SHAPE UP:
Strategies for Health Awareness through Preaching and Empowerment

Dr. Michael Thomas Scott, Sr.

A.A.S, John Tyler Community College, 2002
B.A., Virginia Union University, 1998
M.Div., Virginia Union University, 2001

Mentors
Ricky Woods, D.Min.
Terry Thomas, D.Min.

A FINAL PROJECT DISSERTATION SUBMITTED TO
THE DOCTORAL STUDIES COMMITTEE IN PARTIAL
FULFILLMENT OF THE REQUIREMENTS FOR THE DEGREE
OF DOCTOR OF MINISTRY

UNITED THEOLOGICAL SEMINARY
Dayton, Ohio
December 2006

authorHOUSE®

AuthorHouse™
1663 Liberty Drive
Bloomington, IN 47403
www.authorhouse.com
Phone: 1-800-839-8640

First published by AuthorHouse 4/8/2010

ISBN: 978-1-4520-0698-7 (e)
ISBN: 978-1-4520-0697-0 (sc)

Library of Congress Control Number: 2010904742

Printed in the United States of America
Bloomington, Indiana

This book is printed on acid-free paper.

Table of Contents

ABSTRACT

SHAPE UP:
STRATEGIES FOR HEALTH AWARENESS THROUGH
PREACHING AND EMPOWERMENT

by

Michael Thomas Scott, Sr.
United Theological Seminary, 2006

Mentor
Ricky Woods, D.Min.
Terry Thomas, D.Min.

The objective of this project was to increase the level of health awareness within Jerusalem Baptist Church, Temperanceville, Virginia and to provide a focus group the tools needed to change lifestyle habits resulting in a positive influence upon their health. This was addressed by implementing a forty-day "health awareness season" which included: a nutrition seminar, three relevant sermons, a wellness bible study, and a fast. The participants took the "National Health Test" before and after the intervention and the results revealed that 54% improved. Overall, the project produced a positive impression upon the rural congregation regarding the importance of health.

Acknowledgements

First and foremost I must give all praise and glory to God for enabling and empowering me to commence and complete this work for the health, wellness, and betterment of humankind. Truly with God, "all things are possible."

I would like to acknowledge my mentors, Dr. Ricky Woods and Dr. Terry Thomas for your guidance, direction, support, and words of wisdom. The time that I have spent with you developing this doctoral project has been well spent and the many "nuggets" of inspiration shared are priceless.

To all of the Woods-Thomas "Preaching and Leadership" scholars, I have learned so much from you, just listening, observing, and admiring the unique way that God uses each of you in global leadership and the ministry of the Gospel of Jesus Christ. Special thanks to my peer associate, Pastor Marvin Charlet of Brooklyn, New York for lending your "eyes and ears" throughout this process and for the wonderful health links and websites.

To my professional associates, Ronnie E. Holden, Ed.D., Henry Brown, D.Min., Joan Wharton, D.Min., Alfred S. Beebe, Ph.D., and Kenneth Annan, Ph.D., for your willingness to share of your time, experience, and resources. Special appreciation to Pauline Milbourne and Susan O'Brien of the Accomack County Extension Office of Accomac, Virginia for conducting the health seminar.

I also would like to acknowledge Dr. Bennie L. Smith and my colleagues at Bennie Smith Funeral Home, for making it possible for me to work and attend school simultaneously. It was not easy, but it was worth it!

Much love and appreciation to the officers and members of the Jerusalem Baptist Church of Temperanceville, Virginia, a ministry that is truly one of the best kept secrets on the Eastern Shore of the Commonwealth of Virginia. May you continue to be "the Church on the Shore for People on the Grow!"

Finally, to my loving, devoted, and supportive wife, Lady Tamara T. Scott, for the countless hours of reviewing and editing this work. "May you continue to prosper and be in health even as your soul prospers."

DEDICATION

I DEDICATE THIS DOCTOR OF MINISTRY Final Project Dissertation to my grandparents, for inspiring me to make progress everyday. I also dedicate this work to my parents, Kevin and Shirley Baker and Edward and Belinda Waples, for your love and continued support in all of my ministry endeavors. I dedicate this work to my loving and supportive family, my wife Lady Tamara T. Waples-Scott, my three children Trinity M. Scott, Morgan T. Scott and Michael T. Scott II. Finally, I dedicate this Doctor of Ministry project to countless the individuals throughout the Delmarva Peninsula and the United States of America as a whole. May you realize that God's desire for humanity is that we live a healthy, prosperous, and abundant life.

INTRODUCTION

THIS WORK WAS BIRTHED IN response to a great need within the rural church in the 21st Century. As the writer did a careful analysis of the Jerusalem Baptist Church of Temperanceville, Virginia, in collaboration with context associates, mentors, and professional associates, a ministry project was implemented to address a crucial and critical issue: the need for health awareness. It was evident that many of the officers, leaders, and members of this particular rural ministry were unequipped and unprepared to do ministry effectively in the church and the community because of unhealthy habits and lifestyles. Though the church has a legacy steeped in a rich history of tradition and heritage, the survival of the rural church could be threatened by the church's lack of acknowledgement that God desires that all would "prosper and be in health even as the soul prospers."

The model of ministry to be addressed will seek to raise the level of health awareness among rural church leadership in the 21st Century. The days are gone where individuals can eat whatever they want, however they want, without exercising and taking care of their body, soul, and spirit. The health awareness ministry model to be explored in this document shall focus on the need for the rural church in particular, to raise the issue of holistic health and wellness.

The reader of this document shall see that the writer has attempted to increase the level of health awareness and change the unhealthy habits and lifestyles of rural congregants by combining information, inspiration, and invoke implementation.

The focal point of chapter one will concentrate on the many needs within the ministry focus and will then hone in on actual development of the ministry model: community health education and awareness in the local church. The middle section will focus on the context in which the project was implemented, including a detailed history of the Jerusalem Baptist Church and a general overview of the membership and ministry demographics. The final portion of the first chapter will present a brief spiritual autobiography of the writer, highlighting the writer's own spiritual development and how that has influenced this writing and the ministry project as a whole.

The second chapter will offer a brief synopsis of the literary works that the writer deems necessary to the development of the ministry project. Four primary resources were selected by the writer, and expounded upon to demonstrate a familiarity with the leading authorities and experts in the field of health and health awareness. This chapter will also inform and introduce the reader to the foundational framework of the primary means by which the ministry project will be implemented: the preaching. The writer will expound upon other pertinent literary works in the field of homiletics to further demonstrate a familiarity with leading experts in that field.

The third chapter presents the material that undergirds the entire premise of the ministry project. This chapter will provide a framework for the reader to grasp an adequate understanding of the theological, historical, and biblical foundation upon which the rural church leaders would be equipped and empowered through health awareness.

The fourth chapter will simply describe the method and the design of the health awareness ministry project which was implemented at the Jerusalem Baptist Church. The intervention or treatment applied to the context will be defined and described as well as the instrumentation to be used upon the participants of the ministry model.

The fifth chapter will attempt to reveal the results of the model after it was implemented within the given context. The analysis of the data will be presented as well as a few graphs and charts of illustrative purposes. This chapter will also offer the reader a report of the positive and negative results of the model and its effect upon the context as a whole.

The sixth chapter will offer the writer's own theological and practical reflections on the field experienced discussed in chapter five. The writer will then discuss a few suggestions and recommendation for future research within this field of study. This chapter will provide an overall summary of the ministry project including its successes and failures. This final chapter will serve as a conclusion to the document.

CHAPTER ONE

Ministry Focus

IN A RAPIDLY CHANGING WORLD of modern science, advanced technology, and the information age, many rural churches within America are drastically failing to face the many challenges of effective leadership within the 21st century. It is evident that the rural church, particularly within many African-American communities, is not equipped or prepared to provide the next level of ministry to a world in desperate and dire need of Divine direction and deliverance. As more individuals migrate from the inner cities and urban centers of society into the suburban and rural areas of the countryside, there is a tremendous ministry opportunity for the rural churches within these communities. It is extremely unfortunate that there is a lack of leadership, commitment, and understanding, in the areas of worship, educational ministries, technology, evangelism, community outreach and church growth within the rural ministry context. Preston Robert Washington, pastor of Harlem's Memorial Baptist Church, in his discussion on the renewal of the black church states that, "At the threshold of the twenty-first century, probably the most important question facing the pilgrim people called Afro-Americans is, Will the black church survive? This is not simply a rhetorical question; the church is the single most prominent and important institution in the black community. It is both terrifying and challenging to realize that as the church goes, so goes the community, the nation, and in large measure, the world."[1] The African-American religious community is in need of restoration and renewal, particularly within the rural context of ministry, if effective transformation is to be brought about within the hearts and minds of the people.

Transformative Worship That Informs

One of the main challenges within the ministry focus of the rural church, is that a large portion of the congregants have lost sight of the true mission and primary purpose of the church: the worship of God through Christ. Transformative worship is an integral component to the concept of twenty-first century ministry and leadership. "One of the most important dimensions of the church's ministry is the experience of worship."[2] With all of the challenges and obstacles that life in the twenty-first century will inevitably bring, people need to worship and experience a God that can and will empower them for leadership in every aspect of their personal lives. "The point of prophetic worship is to place people in touch with those transformative elements of meaning which give life new direction, purpose, vitality and strength."[3] It is a sad commentary that many rural churches continue to practice worship methodologies that are ineffective in reaching the needs of people. There is a lack of holistic ministry within the worship experiences of many rural churches,

---

1   Preston Robert Washington, *God's Transforming Spirit: Black Church Renewal* (Valley Forge: Judson Press, 1988), 19.
2   Carlyle Fielding Stewart III, *African American Church Growth: 12 Principles for Prophetic Ministry* (Nashville: Abingdon Press, 1994), 55.
3   Ibid, 57.

which often results in a lack of commitment within the congregation and throughout the community. Effective outreach and community involvement is birthed as a result of a genuine love for and worship of God. "Churches often don't grow because their worship services are dry, lifeless, devoid of the passion and enthusiasm for the celebration of life that the Holy Spirit creates."[4] If the rural church is going to do effective ministry in the twenty-first century, the congregants must be open to innovative ideas and approaches toward a worship encounter that addresses the needs of all people within the context, thus opening up the door for new possibilities in the area of community outreach. Dr. James H. Harris, pastor of Second Baptist Church of Richmond, Virginia addresses the issue of worship that will change, transform, touch lives, and provoke Christians to go forth and do something meaningful within the local community, the region, and even perhaps globally:

> The task of worship in the black church is to be true to our heritage and to God. When I look around urban and rural areas, I see people hurting and in trouble. This suggests that preachers and laypersons have an awesome responsibility in trying to do the will of God. We have to construct public worship in a way that will help change society to what we believe God would have it to be.[5]

The twenty-first century worship experience is an encounter that involves the total transformation of heart, mind, body, and soul through Gospel preaching, meaningful music ministry, authentic fellowship, and genuine praise.

---

4   Ibid, 56.
5   James H. Harris, *Pastoral Theology: A Black Church Perspective*, (Minneapolis: Augsburg Fortress Press, 1991), 95-96.

Educational Ministries

The educational ministries within many rural churches can be viewed as destitute due to the lack of participation, planning, and proper preparation. There is a lack of teaching and training going on within the rural ministry, particularly within the African-American church. It doesn't matter how large or small the congregation, there is usually a vast difference in church attendance on Sunday morning services in comparison to Bible Study, pastoral teaching nights, prayer services, and leadership training classes. "Neither Christian education nor education in general is a priority for the majority in the church. We are a preaching-oriented people, who display a marked lack of support for serious Bible study, workshops, seminars, and general training in spiritual and liberation development."[6] Rural ministry is not equipped for the twenty-first century, due to the fact that many churches invest in large and spacious sanctuaries and areas for preaching and worship, neglecting adequate space and facilities for teaching, training, fellowship, and recreation for all ages. "Christian education in the black church, however, is often lacking in structure and overall systematic goals. Because the church has traditionally been considered a worshipping institution, it has often failed to develop proper facilities for educational ministry."[7] Many rural churches are attempting to do ministry with outdated equipment and inadequate facilities. Many rural churches are still using "outhouses" and others don't even have the benefit of hot running water for hand washing and sanitary purposes within the restrooms. There is a great need for classroom and educational space in the rural church. Dr. Susan Johnson cook, president of the Hampton University Minister's

---

6   Ibid, 101-102.
7   Ibid, 103.

Conference asserts that, "I don't think we're called just to build big churches and mega-churches, I think that we're called to make a difference in lives."[8] Dr. James H. Harris asserts that, "the educational ministry of the church must understand its task in broad terms. This means that before we start discussing theology in any form, we need to meet people where they are. Some will first need to be taught to read and write. Yes, there are persons within the black church who cannot do either."[9]

Technological Advancement

The rural ministry is not adequately prepared for twenty-first century ministry without the use of innovation and technology. Yes, even within the rural ministry context, the use of innovative marketing strategies, internet advertising, and computer technology is absolutely necessary for leadership in the twenty-first century. "Unfortunately, many people today still have antiquated notions about the church and find the idea of developing church marketing strategies sacrilegious. The church should not adopt the 'ways of the world' in spreading the gospel, objected one opponent of the idea."[10] Church records and minutes need to be recorded and properly entered into the computer. For years, many rural churches have made it by "word of mouth." But with the availability of technology at ones fingertips and a fast-paced information age, there is no excuse for the church's reluctance to integrate computer technology into the overall ministry of the church. Children and young people should be able to come into the church to get assistance with homework and

---

8   Dr. Susan Johnson Cook, "Breaking Traditions", *Gospel Today*, Volume 15 Issue 7 (September/October 2004) 36.

9   James H. Harris, *Pastoral Theology: A Black Church Perspective*, 104.

10 Carlyle Fielding Stewart III, *African American Church Growth: 12 Principles for Prophetic Ministry*, 124.

tutorial lessons on the computer. Rural churches need websites and email addresses, in order to become effective in reaching countless individuals who are surfing the internet "looking for love in all of the wrong places." Dr Susan Johnson Cook expounds on the issue of technology in the church:

> For many that also means introducing technology into worship. Many of us who are baby boomers did not grow up using computers and being able to web cast, but we have a generation that we are serving that can instantly get a message to one another. So it's important to understand how to use that to the advantage of ministry and not see it as a hindrance, but as a help.[11]

The integration of modern technology into worship and preaching, educational ministries, evangelism and church outreach programs of the rural context of ministry would greatly help empower rural church leadership in the twenty-first century.

Evangelism and Church Growth

Evangelism and church growth also need to be addressed within the focus of rural church ministry. Because of the fact that many rural churches are family oriented, family owned, and/or family operated, church growth is often retarded or does not occur at all. Many rural congregations are just not prepared for 21st century evangelism, church, growth, and community outreach because they often view the church as an "exclusive community." Carlyle Fielding Stewart III states that, "Too often the church excludes people from it fellowship and membership circles by immediately throwing up

---

11   Dr. Susan Johnson Cook, "Breaking Traditions", *Gospel Today*, 36.

membership smoke screens and other hurdles which keep people out rather than inviting them in."[12] Evangelism and outreach should be on the priority list of rural church leaders, because Christ has mandated this within the Great Commission.[13] Interestingly, Preston Robert Washington states, "The making of disciples goes against the grain of most congregations and church leaders. Part of the problem is laziness. It takes time to make a person a committed follower of Jesus Christ."[14] If the rural church is going to survive, particularly within the African American community, there must be a renewing of the mind and a willingness to carry the Message that God's love is for everyone.

> A great tragedy of Christianity today, and a deterrent to black church growth, is the church's failure to invite people to belong to the fellowship of believers. Too often, a church is guided by a "members only" philosophy and fails to challenge people to participate in the celebration of Christ and his Kingdom. The Christian church has been accused of being an elitist institution whose outreach is limited to "card-carrying members." Many stories have been related about the ways church members shut off potential members by everything from being impervious to ideas from new and potential members to "owning a pew" and not allowing visitors to sit there.[15]

Much teaching and training needs to be done within the context of rural ministry, to help congregants see the importance of evangelism

---

12 Carlyle Fielding Stewart III, *African American Church Growth: 12 Principles for Prophetic Ministry*, 117.

13 Matt. 28:19-20

14 Preston Robert Washington, *God's Transforming Spirit: Black Church Renewal*, 70.

15 Carlyle Fielding Stewart III, *African American Church Growth: 12 Principles for Prophetic Ministry*, 117.

and community outreach within the 21st century. Instead of murmuring and complaining about what the local church is lacking, there needs to be a concerted and unified evangelistic effort that is ongoing and effective in it focus. If only each Christian would begin evangelizing within their own homes and with their family members through "relational evangelism", a great transformation could be experienced in the church as a whole.

On the other hand, there are many rural churches that are attempting to do whatever they can to evangelize and grow the church, however, they often go about it using ineffective methods. Preston Robert Washington addresses the issues of churches attempting to assimilate what they have seen white evangelicals such as Rev. Billy Graham and Rev. Jerry Faldwell.

> Another aspect of the problem is the false idea of evangelism that we have witnessed on television or watched in our churches during revival meetings. The call is made to become a Christian. The person comes forward, is voted into membership or signs his or her name to a card or pledge, and that's the end of it. Often the response was forthcoming in the first place because the atmosphere was emotion-packed or pressure-filled by well-meaning family or friends who pushed the candidate forward. But there is no such thing as a "quickie" Christian. A decision for Christ does not inevitably or automatically lead one to become a fully committed believer.[16]

The work of community outreach and church growth is a serious undertaking, and is a vital component within the rural ministry focus. However, a commitment must be made on the part of the local

---

16   Preston Robert Washington, *God's Transforming Spirit: Black Church Renewal*, 70.

church to step out of "the comfort zone" and the "church as usual" ideologies and begin to make disciples and become "fishers of men."[17] Dr. James H. Harris challenges the black church to take evangelism to another level:

> The black church is compelled to become an extroverted institution—one that will take more risks, demand more justice, and force blacks and whites to move beyond personal conversion to community transformation. To do this, it will have to change its focus of ministry. Rather than emulate the privatistic, personal model represented by modern evangelicalism, it needs to hear anew the great commission in Luke 18:29 and Jesus' message of liberation in Luke 4:18.[18]

It sounds political and militant, but it is high time for the rural church to come up, come out, and come into a 21st century role in ministry. This will require channeling the same old Gospel message and mission through effective methodologies that address current issues facing rural American. If rural church leaders are going to be effective in reaching the masses of people that are migrating back home to their roots in search of a more peaceful and prosperous family life, then church must be willing to accept change in order to bring forth communal transformation. Dr. Susan Johnson Cook said, "What we are beginning to do is almost political. You have to listen to people and find out what their needs are and 'ministry' is meeting the needs of the people that are in your context, that you are serving. We respect the tradition and honor the bridges that have brought us over, but we have to use new methods."[19]

---

17   Mark 1:17
18   James H. Harris, *Pastoral Theology: A Black Church Perspective*, 35.
19   Dr. Susan Johnson Cook, "Breaking Traditions", *Gospel Today*, 36.

Poverty in the Rural Communities

One of the problems is the issue of poverty within the rural community. Within the writer's current context, the church is located in the Northern portion of Accomack County, Virginia, which is ninety-three miles north of Norfolk, Virginia, thirty-nine miles south of Salisbury, Maryland, and approximately 163 miles southwest of Washington, D.C. The primary economic base within Accomack County consists of poultry, farming, and seafood industries. A large majority of the church members, if they are not disabled, are employed as production laborers at the two local poultry plants. In one of the poorest rural counties in the commonwealth of Virginia, one can see that there is a constant struggle with poverty in the black family. A large percentage of families within this rural county and its neighboring county of Northampton, do not even have the modern convenience of indoor plumbing. According to the 2000 U.S. Census report for Accomack County, Virginia: 25.9% of families with children under the age of five years old were reported as living below poverty level. The same report cited that 18% of individuals age 18 and older were living below poverty level, with 15.35 of individual senior citizens age 65 and older living below poverty level.[20] Dr. James H. Harris speaks on poverty and the black church:

> Poverty is real for most black people—now or regularly in the past. The church is responsible for teaching blacks that poverty is a direct result of the greedy, oppressive nature and policies of a society that puts personal gain ahead of community needs. In some cases, it is the result of misguided values and poor work habits, but for the most part, it is directly related

---

20 http://www.factfinder.census.gov, "DP-3 Profile of Economic Characteristics" (2000)

to the economic system. The black church cannot ignore the question of poverty.[21]

There used to be a time when many rural people did not face the problems and challenges often linked to and associated with the urban lifestyle. But time has made a drastic change, and the same conditions that are in the city can be identified within the rural counties. The rural church must take great measures to do some radical ministry in effort to confront these challenges head on.

Development of a Ministry Model:
Community Health Awareness

The writer, in collaboration with mentors and context associates, identified the area of community health educational services with which our rural church leaders can become equipped and empowered to aggressively address relevant issues in 21st century ministry. The problem within this regard is that because of the various factors aforementioned in this document, rural church leaders and members that constitute this rural congregation are currently unprepared and ill-equipped for ministry to the community in the twenty-first century as it relates in particular to the issue of health awareness. First, it is the aim of this ministry model to increase the level of awareness of the importance of the need for ministry in the twenty-first century as it relates to health education within the rural community through the treatment of preaching a brief series of relevant and practical sermons to the leaders and members of this particular rural ministry, Jerusalem Baptist Church. Dr. Terry Thomas asserts:

---

21   Dr. James H. Harris, *Pastoral Theology: A Black Church Perspective*, 78.

> Preaching has always been and always will be the catalyst to motivate people and the source of inspiration to inspire people to continue to move forward when their progress has been impeded or stopped because of some opposing opposition. Leadership in the 21st century must contain an inspiring word to people who do not know how to wait.[22]

Secondly, the writer's objective is to provide a selective focus group within the local community the practical tools needed to change habits that will result in a positive influence upon their health outcomes. This focus group will meet at Jerusalem Baptist Church of Temperanceville, Virginia with the cooperation of church leadership and in partnership with volunteers from the Accomack County Cooperative Extension Agency, the local health department, and the American Cancer Society.

The sociological consideration for this particular ministry model to be addressed is rooted in the fact that healthcare or the lack thereof among minorities within rural communities is experiencing a great decline, particularly within the underserved rural county of Accomack, Virginia. "The increase in health disparities over the past twenty years has been fueled by a complex interplay of lack of access to healthcare, environmental, social, economic, and behavioral factors, action on a history of cultural, income and institutional inequalities."[23] This is clearly a 21st century issue of extreme relevance to the local community that must be addressed by the local church. According to the Virginia Department of Health's Office of Minority

---

22   Dr. Terry Thomas, "An Exploration into the Task of Leadership", a lecture given during United Theological Seminary Peer Seminar.
23   Office of Minority Health (OMH), Executive Summary of the Strategic Plan for April 1, 2004-April 1, 2009, 3.

Health Report for 2002, "the major causes of death for all racial and ethnic groups were heart disease and cancer."[24]

> In 1985, the United States Secretary of Health and Human Services empanelled a Task Force on Minority Health to review the available data and assess the health status of minority Americans. The task force identified six causes of death as collectively accounting for more than 80 percent of the excess death and mortality for African Americans or Blacks and other minority groups. These were cancer, asthma, heart disease and stroke, chemical dependency, diabetes, intentional and unintentional injuries and infant mortality. The task force also discerned that minorities experience significantly poorer health outcomes when compared to their white counterparts.[25]

In addition to these findings, the Virginia Department of Health specifically identifies the Eastern Shore of Virginia, which includes both Accomack and Northampton counties as grant-funded targeted areas because of the large population of underserved and uninsured rural minorities. Sixty percent of adults over age 18 were cited as being overweight in 1998 and 28% of adults over age 18 were cited as being obese within the health district of Virginia's Eastern Shore.[26] The culmination of this ministry model project includes collaboration with the Grayland Baptist Church of Richmond, Virginia which donated (3) three computers to the Jerusalem Baptist Church. The three computers will be used to increase the level of health awareness through the utilization of the American Cancer Society's and other

---

24 Virginia Department of Health, 2002 Minority Health Report, www.ddg. state.va.us/primcare/minority/data/data.asp, 1.
25 Office of Minority Health (OMH), Executive Summary of the Strategic Plan for April 1, 2004-April 1, 2009, 3.
26 Virginia Department of Health, "PHHS Grant-funded Target Areas-Eastern Shore", www.vdh.state.va.us/health/recordstats.asp

pertinent health organizational software for rural church and community members. The software was installed in collaboration with the local HBCU, the University of Maryland Eastern Shore of Princess Anne, Maryland. The usage of the computers introduces the latest 21st century innovation and technology within the church while equipping rural church leadership to do community outreach through health awareness.

The Context

The context where the ministry model was implemented is Jerusalem Baptist Church in Temperanceville, Virginia. Jerusalem Baptist Church is located at 10011 Jerusalem Road, Temperanceville, Virginia, which is apart of local region known as the "Eastern Shore." Jerusalem Baptist church currently consists of a membership that is totally African-American in population. The church is a traditional Baptist ministry, affiliated regionally with the Baptist General Convention of Virginia and locally with the Eastern Shore of Virginia Maryland Baptist Association. Functioning primarily within the rural ministry context, this church is rooted and grounded in a rich history, heritage, and tradition.

In 1861, America was torn apart by a great Civil War, testing on the field of battle whether this nation or any nation could long endure, half slave and half free. On April 9, 1865, the war came to a bloody and bitter end. The African American person was liberated from slavery after nearly three hundred years of oppression. After the slaves were freed, they began to organize churches where they could worship God.

Log Chapel was the first African American church in the northern part of Accomack County, Virginia. However, Log Chapel could not effectively minister to the needs of the people because the distance was far too great and travel in those days was very poor. There was a great need to establish a church in each local community.

"Itinerant black preachers tramped dusty back roads throughout the South, telling Bible stories, and stomping hope into the hearts of the people."[27] The Temperanceville, Virginia area was blessed to have a man sent from God whose name was Jimmie Cluff, a former slave and Civil War veteran. The Reverend Jimmie Cluff was a man of determination and undying faith. He organized a group of people in Temperanceville who called themselves "the Jerusalem Baptist Church." They did not have a building or sanctuary to worship in, so Reverend Cluff held worship experiences under a makeshift tent. Church records indicate that one dark night a storm destroyed his tent. Reverend Cluff then walked up and down the roads, in and around the Temperanceville area selling eggs, butter, and other products of agriculture in effort to raise money to build a church. It was on the twenty-first day of February in 1878, Reverend Cluff and his church members purchased land from Mr. Albert S. Matthews and his wife Mrs. Anna S. Matthews for the purpose of erecting a church edifice.

Reverend Cluff, also served as a traveling pastor to other local Baptist churches in the neighboring communities of New Church, Jenkins Bridge, and Chincoteague Island, all located within the northern portion of Accomack County. Interestingly, Reverend Cluff resigned from the Jerusalem pulpit shortly after the edifice was constructed and was succeeded as pastor by Reverend Perham. Due to conflict, Reverend Perham also resigned as pastor, and the church again sought the leadership of Reverend Cluff. This time Reverend Cluff remained the pastor until the burden of many years had taken

---

27 Samuel DeWitt Proctor, *The Substance of Things Hoped for: A Memoir of African-American Faith*, (New York: G.P. Putnam's Sons, 1995), 6.

their toll. He eventually retired when he was old and well stricken with age.

After the leadership of Reverend Cluff, the church called Reverend Thomas Byrd to the pastorate. After the Byrd administration, the church called the reverend Thomas Turlington. Reverend Turlington was a courageous leader who touched the lives of many people. It was during the Turlington administration that the church was destroyed by fire. Reverend Turlington and his congregation came together and built the church's present edifice. After Reverend Turlington's dynamic leadership came to an end, the church was led by the following ministers, the Rev. Elijah Bowers, Rev. Carrington, Rev. Henderson, and the Rev. Benjamin Burton.

During the Burton administration, the church moved progressively forward. The church parsonage was constructed in the 1950's, the church was renovated, restrooms were installed, the former Jerusalem one-room school house was connected to the edifice to serve as the fellowship hall, new pews were purchased, and the Word of God was preached to the souls of humanity. Due to an internal struggle, Reverend Burton resigned from the pulpit.

Late in 1970, when the church family wandered without a shepherd, many prayers were offered up to God for a new leader. The Reverend Edward Leroy Bruce was called and elected to serve as pastor. The church found Reverend Bruce to be a powerful and prolific preacher with character and great skill. Rev. Bruce was the first seminary trained minister to serve the church. He exposed the church to prominent ministers on the national level during revivals and church crusades. He served as president of the National Alumni Association of Virginia Seminary of Lynchburg, Virginia and as Moderator of the Eastern Shore of Virginia Maryland Baptist Association. During the twenty-seven years of the Bruce administration, the church moved forward by the Spirit of the Lord. The church was renovated, the church building was bricked in1982-83, new carpet was purchased, heat and air-conditioning was installed, an educational wing was constructed, and the Word of god was preached causing many souls to be added to the kingdom. Reverend Bruce died in December of 1997, nearly a few weeks after the church voted to give him a new white robe and a salary increase.

The church family then besought the Lord for a pastor after "God's own heart" to preach, teach, and prepare God's people for the new millennium. In June of 1999, the Reverend Michael Thomas Scott accepted the call to become the tenth pastor of Jerusalem Baptist Church.[28]

Overview of the Church Membership and Ministry

A review of the church records indicates that the church has grown from an active membership of thirty-five to nearly two hundred and twenty-five.[29] An additional eight o'clock contemporary service was implemented to accommodate church growth on Sunday mornings. The church is currently in a period of transition from being a church heavily populated and primarily dominated by senior citizens to an even mixture of youth and young adults. The congregation is also experiencing growth in the areas of "families" joining the church such as married couples and well-established individuals. Church growth in the rural context is very significant in that according to the historical analysis, many rural congregations were established to serve the local community only through the one-room school,

---

28 Historical Sketch of the Jerusalem Baptist Church, Temperanceville, Virginia.

29 Attendance roster of the Jerusalem Baptist Church, Temperanceville, Virginia.

the place of worship for local Black citizens, and the local cemetery for Black burials. A small percentage of the church members are employed as administrators or white-collared professionals such as school teachers, guidance counselors, comptrollers, and school administrators. For the most part, there is a high rate of illiteracy within the entire county due to the poor conditions in the educational system. Due to the rate of illiteracy on Virginia's Eastern Shore, not many of the older members can read the Bible, but they do know the God of the Bible as articulated to them through oral tradition in the Sunday School ministry and Sunday morning sermons.

Spiritual Development

The writer was born in Dover, Delaware on the 31st of August, the eldest son of Kevin S. and Shirley Scott Baker. The writer received most of his early childhood educational experiences within the Delaware public school system. In reflection, it is evident to the writer that God's hands were upon him even at an early age. Growing up as an only child for nearly fifteen years, he spent many hours alone, so he thought. The truth is that he was far from being alone because God was with him. The writer went to great lengths to be loved and acknowledged by those that were around. There was a call from God upon his life for ministry even in elementary school, but like many, he chose to run from it. In effort to receive acceptance, the writer often misbehaved in school which led to one troublesome experience after another. The writer's mother enrolled him in an African American religious private school for one year. That was all that he needed to get on the right track. He learned more about God, self, and the history of African-American heritage than he had ever heard in his seven years of being in public school. The writer and his mother lived in the local project apartments in Dover. This was his first exposure to poverty, violence, crime, and domestic and drug abuse. The writer often went to church on Sundays with his grandmother.

Under the leadership of the late Rev. Dr. James Hazel Williams, the writer's family gathered at the Union Baptist Church in Dover, Delaware for worship, fellowship, and spiritual renewal. The writer received much of his initial Christian training and exposure at Union Baptist. After the death of Dr. Williams, the first ministerial influence in the writer's life, the church wandered in the wilderness for a few years and many of its members left and moved on to other church.

The writer's mother became a member of the Calvary Baptist Church also in Dover. She became very active within the church and began to establish a meaningful relationship with God under the leadership of the pastor, the Rev. Richard M. Avant. Late one Wednesday evening after Bible Study and Prayer Service at Calvary, the writer told his mother that he wanted to have a relationship with God and that he truly desired salvation. The deacons prayed with him and led him to Christ. He was later baptized and received the right hand of Christian fellowship.

Up to this point, the writer had been so busy trying to be accepted by peers that he did not fully comprehend that God was calling him to a life of leadership and service. The writer joined the Youth Choir and eventually became the organist of the choir. He served for two years as president of the Junior Ushers Ministry and eventually became a Deacon-In-Training. At the age of thirteen, the writer expressed an interest in working in the funeral industry. He got a part-time job during the summer months working as a funeral home attendant at the Young's Funeral Home, Milford, Delaware. While in high school, the writer made preparations to attend mortuary school after graduation in order to become a fully licensed mortician. One day while working in the funeral home, the writer injured his back while lifting a casket. This incident was only a mere indication of something far more serious. The writer was diagnosed with scoliosis of the spine and underwent corrective surgery at the A.I. DuPont Children's Hospital in Wilmington, Delaware. While at home in recovery, he missed an entire semester of school and spent countless hours in contemplation. It seemed as if God was revealing to him that he needed to go ahead and do what he had been born to do in the first place, preach God's word. After reading the biblical text found in Jeremiah 1:5-11, the writer received boldness and courage to share with his pastor and others the desire to acknowledge his calling and purpose in life. It was clearly revealed that God had a plan for the writer's life and that everything that had happened previously was in preparation for the mission and ministry that God had in store. At that moment, the writer knew that he was neither an accident, nor was he destined to be a failure or a follower, but God had chosen him for leadership.

> God never does anything accidentally, and [God] never makes mistakes. [God] has a reason for every-thing [God] creates. Every plant and every animal was planned by god and every person was designed with a purpose in mind.[30]

Upon graduating from high school, the writer decided to apply to college. The writer's pastor, Rev. Dr. Richard M. Avant suggested enrollment in Virginia Union University in Richmond, Virginia. The writer's family had very little financial resources to assist in funding his educational pursuits. Through the providential grace of God, the writer was able to secure the finances that were needed to matriculate and remain in college. He worked part-time as a church

---

30   Rick Warren, *The Purpose Driven Life: What On Earth Am I Here For?* (Grand Rapids: Zondervan, 2002), 23.

organist at the Fountain Baptist Church in Richmond, Virginia. He participated in the undergraduate ministerial alliance, served as secretary of the Student Government Association, and as treasurer and chaplain of Alpha Phi Alpha Fraternity, Inc. (Gamma Chapter). Working diligently to complete his undergraduate studies, he attended summer sessions and often took twenty-one credit hours per semester. He finished his undergraduate degree requirements in three years and immediately enrolled in the Samuel DeWitt Proctor School of Theology at Virginia Union.

While in seminary, the writer served as a student intern and eventually as a Minister to the Youth at the Grayland Baptist Church in Richmond, Virginia under the pastoral leadership of Dr. Clifton Whitaker, Jr. This was great time of preparation for the pastoral ministry, which the writer always believed was the area that God was leading him into. The writer traveled with Dr. Ralph Reavis, to study for two weeks at the Overseas Missions Study Center on the campus of Yale University Divinity School in New Haven, Connecticut. Although he took advantage of most opportunities for enrichment, it was a constant struggle to remain in seminary due to financial hardship. In effort to complete his seminary studies without applying for excessive student loans, the writer worked the "graveyard shift" on odd jobs as a tuxedo tailor, dry cleaning assistant, and a security guard for motion pictures, just to make ends meet.

The writer accepted the call to serve as the tenth pastor of the Jerusalem Baptist Church in Temperanceville, Virginia in June 1999. The writer prayed long and hard for an opportunity to exercise God-given gifts, talents, and abilities while leading the people of God. It is the belief of the writer that God answered his prayers and continues to sustain him in the midst of twenty-first century ministry challenges in a traditional Baptist rural congregation.

On September 30, 2000, the writer married his high school sweetheart and soul mate, the former Tamara T. Waples, and God has blessed their union time and time again. Together, they opened Mike's Religious Gift Shoppe, a Christian bookstore in Pocomoke City, Maryland. The writer supported his wife, a former high school English teacher, in the publishing of her first book and the establishment of a publishing and editing business. The writer's wife supported him through completion of his mortuary education and training in effort to become a licensed mortician. It is their vision to establish their very own funeral service business. God has blessed them with two beautiful daughters, Trinity and Morgan that offer a great source of strength, stability, and support in the midst of ministry triumphs and challenges.

God has allowed for the writer to grow up from humble beginnings in order to return to humble beginnings in ministry. The writer had to experience a certain degree of poverty, pain, and personal crisis in order to preach the liberating Gospel of Christ unto those who have been held captive to the same perils and challenges in the rural setting.

The State of the Art in This Ministry Model

THE FOCAL POINT OF CHAPTER Two will be to examine the key resources that are relevant to equipping and empowering rural church leaders in 21st century ministry through health awareness. A narrative exposition of how these resources prove beneficial to the development of this ministry model will be exhibited. The writer will identify significant concepts and other models of ministry that have greatly informed and influenced this particular ministry focus. This chapter will provide a demonstration of the writer's familiarity with the literature and resources directly related to the issue of raising the level of health awareness in the local rural congregation, particularly through the ministry of preaching.

Resource Review

Five primary resources have been consulted for the purpose of the development of this particular ministry model. Dr. George H. Malkmus' work entitled, *Why Christians Get Sick*[31], is a product

---

31 Dr. George H. Malkmus, *Why Christians Get Sick*, (Shippensburg, PA: Treasure House, 1997).

of one man's personal experience with a colon cancer diagnosis at the age of 42. Dr. Malkmus, an ordained minister, dedicated his entire life to biblical and scientific research to raise the level of health awareness and education particularly within the church. Jordan Rubin, who also suffered more than eighteen life-threatening diseases and health conditions at the age of nineteen, shares in his book, *The Great Physician's Rx for Health and Wellness: Seven Keys to Unlock Your Health Potential*[32], how he overcame his sickness, obtained optimum health, and seeks to increase awareness of God's ideal health plan. Rubin's book relating to health and wellness from a Christian perspective, offers practical tools needed to live a long, prosperous, healthy and abundant life. Some of the practical tools received from this book for the development of this particular ministry project include: information on fasting and toxic relief, fitness and advance hygiene techniques, deadly emotions and stress, healthy recipes and nutritional guides. Reginald Cherry, M.D. speaks to the issue of spirituality and health from a Christian physician's perspective in his work entitled, *Healing Prayer: God's Divine Intervention in Medicine, Faith, and Prayer*[33]. *Walking in the Light: A Jewish-Christian Vision of Healing and Wholeness*[34] by Bruce G. Epperly and Lewis D. Solomon proved to provide a plethora of holistic concepts from a Judeo-Christian theological standpoint. Also, a wealth of practical information was gleaned from a lecture entitled, "The Role of the Church in Health"[35], delivered by Dr. Terry

32 Jordan Rubin with David Remedios, M.D., *The Great Physician's Rx for Health and Wellness: Seven Keys to Unlock Your Health Potential*, (Nashville: Thomas Nelson Publishers, 2005).

33 Reginald Cherry, M.D., *Healing Prayer: God's Divine Intervention in Medicine, Faith, and Prayer*, (Nashville: Thomas Nelson Publishers, 1999).

34 Bruce G. Epperly and Lewis D. Solomon, *Walking in the Light: A Jewish-Christian Vision of Healing and Wholeness*, (St. Louis: Chalice Press, 2004).

35 Terry Mason, M.D., "The Role of The Church in Health" (lecture delivered at the Doctor of Ministry Intensive Seminar at United Theological Seminary,

Mason, M.D., Commissioner of Health for the City of Chicago and Assistant Professor of Urology at the University of Illinois.

The issue of health awareness within the ministry of the church must be addressed with more commitment, consistency and creativity now more than ever before. More initiative should be taken within the church to help parishioners and members of the local community look at holistic health and wellness from all angles. Historically, health and spirituality have often gone hand in hand. According to Dr. Reginald Cherry, "At present, more than 325 studies have been done on the role of 'spirituality and health'."[36] This is remarkable considering the fact that:

> The majority of doctors were so focused on the physical aspects of sickness and disease that they failed to consider the mental or spiritual part of the people they treated. Many physicians went so far as to suspect that patients who openly believed in spiritual things—who saw God as a personal Being who was interested in their health and welfare—were mentally deranged."[37]

However, the concern of the writer is not the addressing of the health awareness issue, but the manner in which it is addressed, particularly within the rural context of the African-American church. Dr. Terry Mason asserts, "unfortunately, health has taken too much of a backseat in all of our churches. That has got to be apart of the mission of the church to make sure that we not only steward over the spiritual health of the church, but the physical health of the church as well."[38]

Dayton, Ohio on 25 January 2006).

36 Reginald Cherry, M.D., *Healing Prayer: God's Divine Intervention in Medicine, Faith, and Prayer*, 21.

37 Ibid, 9.

38 Dr. Terry Mason, "The Role of the Church in Health".

> Christians, including pastors, evangelists, and missionaries, need to change their thinking concerning sickness and health! They need to start questioning whether their present diet and lifestyle will produce sickness or superior health! A mind open to new thoughts is an absolute necessity if superior health is to be obtained."[39]

The commitment to health awareness should begin within the church and through church leadership. The reality of the matter is that it is tremendously difficult for pastors and church leaders to effectively minister to others about spirituality or holistic health concerns when they are unhealthy themselves. Dr. George H. Malkmus, a full-time pastor and teacher with a once thriving ministry in upstate New York, found himself to be ineffective in ministry due to "burn-out" and "stress" which ultimately led to a diagnosis of colon cancer in the prime of his life at the age of forty-two. This traumatic event happened shortly after he had to watch his mother suffer and die from the same type of cancer. Bruce G. Epperly and Lewis D. Solomon note:

> The traditional professions—medicine, law, and ministry—whose purpose is to nurture and restore order, balance, and health to the world, are now diseased. The evidence of professional dysfunction is everywhere—in rising burnout, stress-related illness, and addiction among professions; in lawsuits and accusations of professional misconduct; in the proliferation of minor forms of boundary violations; in divorce, family alienation, and loss of vitality and vision.[40]

---

39 Dr. George H. Malkmus, *Why Christians Get Sick*, 113-114.
40 Bruce G. Epperly and Lewis D. Solomon, *Walking in the Light: A Jewish-Christian Vision of Healing and Wholeness*, 75.

Dr. Malkmus states, "After watching my own mother go through this terrible ordeal, I was determined not to follow the conventional cancer treatments in my own body. So I searched for and found an alternative…nutrition and a changed lifestyle!"[41] At present, this question of whether to utilize traditional and conventional treatment methods versus non-traditional alternatives is highly controversial. This was particularly revealed with the death of civil rights activist, Coretta Scott King, whose family decided to take her to Mexico for alternative treatments for ovarian cancer.

For all practical purposes, this particular ministry model will focus upon awareness, prevention, and nutrition. Research has repeatedly revealed that individuals need to focus upon healthy eating habits and nutrition, if there is going to be any improvement with health outcomes, particularly in the United States of America. Dr. Malkmus states, "The food presently being consumed and the lifestyle that is being followed is slowly destroying the health and vitality of our great nation, including the Christian community! Various forms of sickness and disease are consuming a larger and larger part of our energy, time, money, and emotions!"[42] Dr. Terry Mason holds that, "Our weapons of mass destruction are our knives and forks and the stuff we put into our mouths."[43] Dr. Reginald Cherry suggests:

> Stopping disease before it starts is much more effective and beneficial than seeking to recover from sickness and repair the body from the ravages of disease. Overeating plays a role in many modern-day diseases and ailments. Organs do not function well when the body is overnourished, obese, and overloaded. Or if

---

41   Dr. George H. Malkmus, *Why Christians Get Sick*, 5.
42   Ibid, 116.
43   Dr. Terry Mason, "The Role of the Church in Health".

the wrong kinds of foods are eaten, the body may not receive the essential nutrients for good health.[44]

Dr. Terry Mason, in his lecture, alluded to the fact that currently the number one cause of cancer and cancer deaths in America is tobacco. However, "adult diets and obesity will soon overtake cigarette smoking as the number one cause of preventable deaths in America. Tobacco, obesity, and sedentary lifestyles contribute to over 800,000 deaths per year."[45] It is evident that there needs to be an attitudinal change of lifestyle if there is going to be any affect upon the health disparities in America. Dr. Reginald Cherry states:

> The foods we eat have a dramatic impact on our health. We should not be amazed, therefore, that six of the ten leading causes of death in this country today are directly linked to our nutritional intake, and this includes diseases such as cardiovascular disease (heart disease and stroke), cancer, lung disease, pneumonia, and diabetes. Americans spend more on diet plans, weight reduction programs, pills, shots, and exercise equipment than the entire national budget of many countries. Isn't it ironic that Americans in reality are malnourished, overfed, obese, and nutrient starved? Many Americans have the same nutritional problems as people in Third World countries, but to the opposite extreme![46]

This ministry focus is grounded in a commitment to combat disease and infirmity within the church and the community by disseminating information that will produce positive healthy lifestyles

---

44 Dr. Reginald Cherry, M.D., *Healing Prayer: God's Divine Intervention in Medicine, Faith, and Prayer,* 49.

45 Dr. Terry Mason, "The Role of the Church in Health."

46 Dr. Reginald Cherry, M.D., *Healing Prayer: God's Divine Intervention in Medicine, Faith, and Prayer,* 39-40.

and choices through nutrition and healthy eating. Dr. D. M. Heigsted, distinguished Professor of Nutrition at the Harvard School of Public Health states:

> Ischemic heart disease, cancer, diabetes and hyperten-
> sion are the diseases that kill us. They are epidemic in
> our population. We cannot afford to temporize. We
> have an obligation to inform the public of the current
> state of knowledge and to assist the public in making
> the correct food choices. To do less is to avoid our
> responsibility.[47]

A careful review of literature and studies related to health promotion and awareness indicate that what an individual eats determines the outcome of their health. Most research suggests that a consistent diet of healthy foods, including fruits and vegetables, can lead to positive holistic healthy outcomes. Dr. Terry Mason holds that "The problem with the American diet is that it's meat-centered. If we focus on fruits and vegetables and not so much what comes from animals, this is our prescription to get us out of the problem that we are in."[48] If there is going to be a reversal of the health disparities that too often lead to death within the African-American community, the consistent consumption of nutritious foods must be stressed. Dr. Reginald Cherry says:

> I believe a crucial key to healing and health is one's
> diet. What you eat, good or bad, to a significant ex-
> tend determines the ultimate state of your health and
> well-being. After years of studying the human body
> from the standpoint of finding ways to avoid sickness

---

47 Dr. D. M. Heigsted, (A press conference held at the Dirkson Senate Office Bldg. Room 457 Harvard School of Public Health, Boston, Massachusetts, on 14 January 1977).

48 Dr. Terry Mason, "The Role of The Church in Health".

and prevent disease, I am convinced that our choice of foods—what we eat and what we avoid—is the most potent program for good health that is within our control.[49]

A key component of this ministry project has been informed by *Body and Soul: A Celebration of Healthy Eating and Living*[50], a relevant model of ministry geared primarily toward the African American church which promotes the consumption of more fruits and vegetables. "Two programs were combined to create *Body and Soul:* "Black Churches United for Better Health" and "Eat for Life." These programs were conducted in churches of various sizes and denominations. The churches were located in urban, suburban, and rural areas. Regardless of the location or size, each of these faith-based programs was highly successful in helping church members eat more fruits and vegetables."[51] Jordan Rubin states, "Fruits and vegetables, when consumed at optimal amounts have been shown in countless studies to protect us against the ravages of heart disease, high blood pressure, cancer, diabetes, and almost every killer disease common to modern men and women."[52] *Body and Soul* stresses the importance of using creative methods to get African American church members to consume five to nine servings of fruits and vegetables per day. Research suggests that Americans as a whole are lacking significant nutrients because of the fact that fruits and vegetables

---

49 Dr. Reginald Cherry, *Healing Prayer: God's Divine Intervention in Medicine, Faith, and Prayer*, 49.

50 *Body and Soul: A Celebration of Healthy Eating and Living: A Guide for Your Church* is a program developed as the result of 10 years of research developed by the National Cancer Institute, American Cancer Society, University of North Carolina, and the University of Michigan.

51 Ibid, 25.

52 Jordan Rubin with David Remedios, M.D., *The Great Physician's Rx for Health and Wellness: Seven Keys to Unlock Your Health Potential*, 88.

are not consumed as consistently as they should be. Jordan Rubin elaborates:

> The average American consumes less than the recommended three-to-five servings a day of "greens" and the most beneficial are the deep green, leafy vegetables. In fact, Americans eat way less than they should when it comes to consuming their green veggies. The United States Department of Agriculture estimates that more than 90% of the population fail to eat five to nine servings of the most beneficial foods that God created on this planet.[53]

It is quite evident that there is a tremendous need for another ministry project relating to health awareness and promotion, particularly within the African American community. However, this particular ministry project focuses upon the creative abilities of the preacher to incorporate the message of healing and health awareness with the Gospel of Jesus Christ. Dr. George H. Malkmus contends:

> There are literally thousands of ministers helping to prepare people to die. But how many are teaching people how to live? How many are teaching people how to live a vibrantly healthy, abundantly happy life so that they will have the energy and health to share Christ, yea, even the health to remain alive to tell the good news.[54]

It is the purpose of this ministry project, to inform the context, which is the local rural congregation of the importance of health awareness, both individually and corporately, through the preachment. Dr. George H. Malkmus further states:

---

53 Ibid, 87.
54 Dr. George H. Malkmus, *Why Christians Get Sick?*, 120.

> In the churches, pastors and Sunday School teachers must include in their teachings, the proper care of the body, "God's Temple!" Our Christian schools and colleges must offer courses that teach the biblical approach to the care of the body, and curriculum must be developed for the classroom!"[55]

This however, is easier said than done. Preaching and teaching with relevancy to such a subject in this 21st century, will require significant preparation on part of the preacher. The clarity and creativity needed to convict and convince the congregation of this imperative issue will necessitate the exposition of relevant preaching resources. With this in mind, the writer will now consider a careful review of relevant concepts as it relates to the area of specialization used to promote this ministry project: preaching.

Preparation for Preaching

It is evident that preaching the Gospel in the 21st century is more than a notion. In fact it is a serious undertaking. Preaching a relevant word in this new millennium will require extensive preparation on the part of the preacher. Gospel preaching that is deliberate, purposeful, and effective comes from great preparation. Preparation is defined as "the action or process of making something ready for use or service or getting ready for some occasion, test, or duty."[56] Preachers in this 21st century should be concerned about the preparatory stages of the preachment as much as the delivery of the sermon. Gospel preaching in this 21st century will necessitate spiritual discipline and

---

55 Ibid, 114.
56 *Merriam-Webster Collegiate Dictionary*, 10th edition, Springfield, Mass (1999), 920.

nourishment of the inner life, homiletical exegesis and study, and some practical points of preparation for relevancy.

Spiritual Discipline & Nourishment of the Inner Life

Dr. Ricky Woods contends that:

> Getting ready to preach does not start with the selection of a text or the development of a thesis, getting ready to preach begins with nurturing an intimate relationship with [the God] whom we proclaim. The demonic temptation in ministry today is not what happens to us or with us in proclamation, but what happens to us before we reach the pulpit.[57]

It is imperative that the preacher develop a spiritually disciplined life. The nourishment of the inner life is a prerequisite to preaching with relevance and effectiveness in the 21st Century. Not only should the preacher take the calling and task of preaching as a serious undertaking, but also the preacher should take it personally. Historically, the early apostolic fathers and mothers of the New Testament had a personal and meaningful relationship with Christ that heavily influenced and informed their ability to proclaim a relevant gospel with great boldness and faith. In John's account of the resurrection, Mary Magdalene was the first to have a personal encounter with the risen Christ. She was so excited when she saw her Lord that she held on to him and would not let go:

> Jesus said to her, "Stop clinging to Me, for I have not yet ascended to the Father; but go to My brethren and say to them, 'I ascend to My Father and your Father,

---

57 Dr. Ricky Woods, "Getting Ready to Preach", lecture presented at United Theological Seminary Preaching and Leadership peer seminar, Baltimore, Maryland, (November 2004).

> and My God and your God.'" Mary Magdalene came,
> announcing to the disciples, "I have seen the Lord,"
> and that He had said these things to her."[58]

Nothing can replace the spiritual benefits and blessings of having a personal relationship with Christ. Calvin Miller, homiletics professor at Southwestern Baptist Theological Seminary asserts, "great preachers are great because they lift Sunday's messages, paragraph by paragraph, from the personal altars of their lives."[59] Great sermons and messages are the direct result of those quiet moments of personal preparation with the Divine all throughout the week. Spiritual discipline within the private life of the preacher is an essential ingredient to preaching sermons that will have an impact on the public. "Great sermons are not born in illustration books but in the needy lives of preachers. Here where the preachers' inwardness is fashioned by yearning and desperation, is the womb of important preaching."[60]

Norman Shawchuck and Roger Heuser identify three key elements of the spirituality of Jesus during his public ministry that could be imitated by today's gospel preachers. First of all, "Jesus carried out his ministry within the context of a small, intimate, covenant community."[61] Upon going forth into public ministry, Jesus chose twelve disciples or followers that would serve with him and for him as a covenant community. He chose these twelve disciples, so that they would be there with Him, even in difficult times. "And from within this community of twelve others, he formed an even

---

58 Jn 20: 17-18 (NAS)
59 Calvin Miller, *Marketplace Preaching: How to Return the Sermon to Where It Belongs,* Grand Rapids: Baker Books, (1995), 11.
60 Ibid, 10.
61 Norman Shawchuck and Roger Heuser, *Leading the Congregation: Caring for Yourself While Serving the People,* Nashville: Abingdon Press, (1993), 46.

more intimate relationship with three [Peter, James, and John]."[62] Every preacher needs relationship, not only with God, but also with other preachers and/or spiritual persons that can serve as a covenant community. "The significance of relationships has been documented by medical research and personal experience. Medical studies show that healthy social contact improves quality of life and may increase a person's lifespan."[63] In following the example of Christ, preachers of the Gospel need a small, intimate network of prayer partners and a support system to share with in preparation. Dr. Ricky Woods in his lecture entitled "Getting Ready to Preach" recommends:

> ...preachers to have prayer partners that are preachers. Persons who understand ministry and the burden as well as the blessing of preaching that will pray with you and for you. Prayer partners also provide a wonderful source of accountability to keep us as preachers from being too busy to pray. [64]

Second, one can learn from the Savior the importance of time management and spiritual centering for holistic ministry:

> Jesus established a rhythm of public ministry and private time. It is clear that Jesus ordered his life and public ministry around a rhythm, a discipline, of moving from public ministry to solitude and prayer. He went *to* ministry from solitude and prayer, and he went *from* ministry to solitude and prayer. Even though he had his community, he continually found those "lonely places" where he was with God alone.[65]

---

62 Ibid, 46.
63 Bruce G. Epperly and Lewis D. Solomon, *Walking in the Light: A Jewish-Christian Vision of Healing and Wholeness*, 53.
64 Dr. Ricky Woods, "Getting Ready to Preach", lecture
65 Norman Shawchuck and Roger Heuser, *Leading the Congregation: Caring for Yourself While Serving the People*, 46-47.

It is imperative to the spiritual life of the preacher, to retreat from the rigors of preaching revivals, church administration, pastoral ministry and leadership, and even one's own family members, to a deserted place of solitude for personal time alone with God. "Health involves an appropriate balance of work and play, and activity and quiet."[66] "Thirdly, Jesus taught by example that six "graces" were vital to his life and ministry: prayer and fasting, the Lord's Supper, the Scriptures, spiritual conversation, and worship in the Temple. These he incorporated into the fabric of his life in order to sustain his ministry."[67]

"First, prayer is the instrument that creates lines of communication between the preacher and God."[68] The preacher should spend time in prayer on a daily basis, not just during the moments prior to proclamation. "Calvin Miller asserts that "our inner life in Christ is the defining work of the spiritual disciplines. Therefore, the preacher ought never to pray merely to empower the sermon. The preacher should pray out of spiritual neediness."[69] According to Dr. Terry Thomas, "the preacher must be a [person] of prayer. Not only must the preacher be a [person] of prayer, the preacher must also be sensitive to the Spirit.[70] In these quiet moments of prayer, one must remain open to the voice of God and fresh revelations for the people of God.

---

66 Bruce G. Epperly and Lewis D. Solomon, *Walking in the Light: A Jewish-Christian Vision of Healing and Wholeness*, 27.

67 Ibid, 47.

68 Dr. Ricky Woods, "Getting Ready to Preach", lecture presented at United Theological Seminary Preaching and Leadership peer seminar, Baltimore, Maryland (November 2004).

69 Calvin Miller, *Marketplace Preaching: How to Return the Sermon to Where It Belongs,* Grand Rapids: Baker Books (1995),8.

70 Dr. Terry Thomas, "From Hunch to Proclamation", lecture presented at United Theological Seminary Preaching and Leadership peer seminar, Hilton Head, South Carolina (March 2005).

The Lord God has given me the tongue of disciples, that I may know how to sustain the weary one with a word. He awakens me morning by morning, He awakens my ear to listen as a disciple. The Lord God has opened my ear and I was not disobedient nor did I turn back. [71]

According to Dr. Frank A. Thomas, "Prayer places us in the posture to discern what God wants to accomplish in the midst of the gathered congregation. God's intention for the sermon can only be accessed through disciplined and fervent prayer."[72] Dr. Ricky Woods states that "prayer has to be scheduled and planned. Every preacher should have a time and place when he/she goes regularly to be alone with God."[73]

Prayer coupled with fasting also makes it easier for the preacher to hear the "voice of the Lord" as recorded in Acts 13:2-3. "Jesus fasted as his final preparation for going public in his ministry. Obviously he felt it important to the work he was to do."[74] Prayer and fasting also helps to discipline the preacher for effectiveness in ministry. In fact, this is what Jesus meant when he spoke to the disciples in Matthew 17:21 in response to why they were unable to cast a demon out of a child. He answered them saying, "But this kind does not go out except by prayer and fasting."[75]

The preacher's participation in the Lord's Supper has a significant and symbolic purpose in the preparation for proclamation. According to Shawchuck and Heuser, "it is striking that as his last free act before

---

71   Isaiah 50:4-5 (NAS)
72   Frank A. Thomas, *They Like To Never Quit Praisin' God: The Role of Celebration in Preaching*, Cleveland: United Church Press (1997), 65.
73   Dr. Ricky Woods, "Getting Ready to Preach", lecture
74   Norman Shawchuck and Roger Huser, *Leading the Congregation: Caring for Yourself While Serving the People*, 47.
75   Matt. 17:21 (NAS)

his terrible passion and death, Jesus chose to eat with his community. He wanted to be remembered by his friends. He also knew that the meal was a healing and restoring event."[76] Dr. Miles Jerome Jones, in his book entitled *Preaching Papers: The Hampton and Virginia Union Lectures*, lifts up the spiritual significance of the Lord's Supper by examining the events that took place on that Maundy Thursday in the upper room. Dr. Jones suggests that there is a connection between the supper, the symbol, and the sermon. Expounding upon the phrase "this is my body"[77], Dr. Miles J. Jones states:

> Perhaps it is at the table as nowhere else we can hear the words that will make us sharers of his real presence in the experiences of our neighborhoods. This is my body, be a part of it and me in the world of daily reality. I know there are times when the preference is to be part of 'my spirit' but the greater need is here; this is my body, the agent of participation in the nitty-gritty of human experience. Go where I would go—to the graveyard and to the wedding feast. Do what I would do; shed a tear in compassion or strike a blow in indignation.[78]

The fourth "spiritual grace" lifted up by Shawchuck and Heuser is the reading of the Scriptures. It is imperative that the preacher takes the time to read the Bible on a daily basis. Jesus had a love for the sacred scriptures. Even as a little boy, Jesus was found by his parents in the Temple sitting at the feet of the scribes and doctors of the law listening to the Scriptures and probing into the Word of God. Preachers should develop a strategic plan of personal study

---

76 Norman Shawchuck and Roger Heuser, *Leading the Congregation: Caring for Yourself While Serving the People*, 47.

77 Matt. 26:26

78 Miles Jerome Jones, *Preaching Papers: the Hampton and Virginia Union Lectures*, (New York: Martin Luther King Fellows Press, 1995), 27.

and devotional time particularly within the Bible. Dr. Ricky Woods expounds on daily bible reading:

> I speak not of the reading for sermons, Bible studies or other presentations to be given which caused the reading, but the reading simply out of a love for the Word of god. Daily Bible reading allows the soul to fill itself from the bread of life and in return can crowd out the distraction that so easily dims the eyes of faith. Most preaching is done from the overflow, i.e., that which comes from the private reserves of the preacher's experiences, context, and scripture readings…Without sufficient storage of the word within us, there will be none to draw up at preaching time.[79]

The blessings of a daily bible reading regimen are too numerous to name. When the preacher spends time contemplating and brooding over the Word of God in daily preparation, the results will be visible upon his or her face upon mounting the pulpit. Dr. Terry Thomas asserts,

> That a constant fresh word from the Lord is the result of working hard in the constant and consistent study of the Word of God. To get a fresh word from God, you have to constantly stay afresh before God with a receptive mind that is eager and ready to receive.[80]

"True preaching comes when the loving heart and the disciplined mind are laid at the disposal of the Holy Spirit."[81]

The fifth spiritual "grace" necessary for the preparation of the preacher is spiritual conversation and meditation. "The Gospels are

---

79 Dr. Ricky Woods, "Getting Ready to Preach"
80 Dr. Terry Thomas, "From Hunch to Proclamation"
81 Haddon W. Robinson, *Biblical Preaching*, (Grand Rapids: Baker Books House, 1980), 25.

filled with serious conversations of a spiritual nature that Jesus had with his twelve disciples, and others who were curious and serious about life's choices."[82] Dr. Ricky Woods asserts, "Meditation calls on us not to do but to reflect and listen. Reflection allows our thoughts to be filtered through the Holy Spirit. In as much as the preaching enterprise begins with [God] and not us, we need to take time to meditate in order to hear."[83] Dr. Woods during his lecture, "Getting Ready to Preach", recommended for preachers to engage in the spiritual journaling to aid in the meditative process. "The journal can help the preacher to be thoughtful and honest in what he or she writes and says to God. The journal might also provide a source for reflection to see how God answered prayer."[84]

Worship is the sixth spiritual "grace" lifted up by Shawchuck and Heuser as essential preparation for preaching and proclamation. It was the custom of Jesus to attend synagogue on a regular basis. Worship is defined as "reverence offered a divine being or supernatural power; also an act of expressing such reverence."[85] Oftentimes the preacher spends countless hours as worship leader and preparing for proclamation, that he or she fails to worship and reverence God on a personal basis. Worship is not limited to what takes place within the confines of the corporate community of Christ. "Worship happens anytime we spend time in praise, adoration, thanksgiving and declaring the glory and worth of God. Worship provides an opportunity for God to disclose [God-self] to the one who worships God."[86] "A religion of survival that facilitates divine power for actions of justice, epitomized in worship, actually empowers worshipers to hear God speak directly

---

82 Norman Shawchuck and Roger Heuser, *Leading the Congregation: Caring for Yourself While Serving the People*, 48.

83 Dr. Ricky Woods, "Getting Ready to Preach"

84 Ibid.

85 *Merriam-Webster's Collegiate Dictionary*, 1365.

86 Dr. Ricky Woods, "Getting Ready to Preach"

to them."[87] "The preacher should take advantage of every opportunity to worship whether that worship is in private with God and self or that worship is in the corporate community of believers where the preacher is not just worship leader but a worship participant."[88] The process of personal preparation in the Spirit, propels one to a biblical passage or pericope that is to be proclaimed to God's people. However, before that passage can be preached, the preacher must undergo the process of exegesis.

Homiletical Exegesis

The process of exegesis is absolutely necessary for relevant preaching in this 21st century. Why is exegesis so essential to the preaching process? "The process of traditional exegesis to discover what the author intended to communicate is the first step in discovering what meaning the Holy Spirit intended in the text. The central question for African American homiletical exegesis is: what meaning (assurance) does the gospel shed on the human condition of suffering through the particular biblical text to be preached?"[89] Exegesis involves "pulling out" or "extracting" from the text those key elements of the original intentions of the author so that the text can then "speak for itself." Margaret Davies asserts: "The art of exegesis lies in elucidating expressions in their appropriate historical context. It attempts to establish the most original reading of the text and to explain variants..."[90] Dr. Terry Thomas in his lecture, "From Hunch to Proclamation" says:

---

87   Melva Wilson Costen, *African American Christian Worship*, (Nashville: Abingdon Press, 1993), 121.
88   Dr. Ricky Woods, "Getting Ready to Preach"
89   Frank A. Thomas, *They Liked to Never Quit Praisin' God*, 67-70
90   R.J. Coggins and J.L. Houlden ed., *A Dictionary of Biblical Interpretation* 1990 edition, (London: SCM Press, 1990), 220-221.

> I have to do an interpretation of the interpretation. I have to try to unfold the implication of the original wording of the text, the work of exegesis. What the text really means is not all what it seems to say to us directly. And what appears to be the meaning of a word in one text does not necessarily carry over into its use in another.[91]

Here, the preacher must spend time with the given text to explicate the hidden meanings within the text, so that he or she is well informed as to what the author's original intent was.

> In such study we can arrive at the various scriptures that might complement or explain the text and focal passage. Again, remember that there is nothing more powerful than letting Scripture speak to scripture. Wherever possible, let other Bible citations speak to, explain, illuminate, and reinforce both the larger context and the focal passage.[92]

Margaret Davies further expounds on exegesis, "The Word suggests a close reading of scriptural texts, explicating terms and sentences, and is often contrasted with 'eisegesis'."[93]

What is eisegesis? Eisegesis is a "modern coinage, by analogy with exegesis, to denote the practice of reading one's own ideas into (Greek *eis*) rather than out of (Greek *ex*) the text of scripture."[94] The temptation of the preacher to force his or her own agenda upon the given text is always present. This must be avoided at all costs, because the text must speak for itself. Again, Dr. Terry Thomas notes, "I have

---

91 Dr. Terry Thomas, "From Hunch to Proclamation"
92 Calvin Miller, *Marketplace Preaching: How to Return the Sermon to Where it Belongs*, 150.
93 R.J. Coggins and J.L. Houlden, ed., *A Dictionary of Biblical Interpretation*, 220-221.
94 Ibid, 187-188.

to be careful that I do not read my personal feelings into my 'hunch'. This statement might find disagreement, but the Bible was not written to us, but for us. We are third party recipients."[95]

In this stage of preparation for preaching with relevancy for health awareness, it is imperative that the text be the focal point of the preacher's concentration. One must be careful in his or her quest for relevancy and effectiveness for today's generation, not to sacrifice the sacredness of the biblical text. Before consulting various commentaries or the internet and other secular sources, the preacher should focus upon the given biblical text. Dr. James H. Harris states:

> In my view, the textuality of the message determines its validity and establishes the message as an authentic sermon rather than a religious speech, a powerful oration, or a spiritual discourse. In its authentic form, the sermon is more than a powerful speech or a moving discourse because it is grounded in the scriptural text.[96]

Once the preacher examines the text as to determine the original meaning and intent of the author, there is yet much work to be done to prepare the sermon for relevancy in the 21st century. "Exegesis, though necessary, is only the first stage in the interpretation of a text."[97] "Exegetical information without meaning leaves hearers participating in an intellectual exercise, but not encountering the text."[98] "After study, prayer, writing, singing, and doing everything else to prepare ourselves for the task of proclamation, our weakness prevents us from being totally ready to preach. However, when it is

---

95 Dr. Terry Thomas, "From Hunch to Proclamation"
96 James H. Harris, *Preaching Liberation*, (Minneapolis: Fortress Press, 1995) 6.
97 R.J. Coggins and J.L. Houlden, *A Biblical Dictionary of Interpretation*, 220.
98 Frank A. Thomas, *They Liked to Never Quit Praisin' God*, 72.

time to preach the gospel of Jesus Christ, 'the spirit helps us in our weakness'."[99]

Practical Points of Preparation

Finally, there are some practical points of preparation for preaching a relevant word. After the preacher has spent time nurturing the inner life and exegeting the biblical text, there are at least three aspects of preparation for effectiveness. First, in this age of technology and information, the preacher should strive to become well-informed before approaching the pulpit. Dr. Terry Thomas calls this phase of preparation, "contemporizing the hunch." In addition to becoming familiar with the biblical text, the preacher must be well-informed in other pertinent areas of life as well. The well-informed preacher, should stay abreast of current events and happenings within today's society by reading local, regional, and national newspapers. The well-informed preacher that seeks to develop his or her effectiveness through relevancy, will consistently view news programs such as "CNN", "MSNBC", and internet sources. The preacher should at least be somewhat familiar with the "bad news" in today's world, so that he or she can effectively communicate the "Good News of Jesus Christ" in response to what people have heard throughout the week. The well-informed preacher will also seek to address subjects that are at the forefront of people's minds in this 21st century. Calvin Miller asserts that there are at least four "instant-interest subjects" in the mentality of today's congregants: security, success, the entrepreneurial mind, and destiny and decision-making."[100] The well-informed preacher will also make it his or her business to attend conferences, seminars, and

---

99 James H. Harris, *Preaching Liberation*, 34.

100 Calvin Miller, *Marketplace Preaching: How to Return the Sermon to Where it Belongs*, 61.

other continuing education events in order to tap into the heartbeat of relevant preaching throughout America, such as the E.K. Bailey Conference on Expository Preaching, the Hampton University Minister's Conference, and the John Malcus Ellison Conference at Virginia Union University to name a few.

Next, in addition to being well-informed, the preacher should be well-prepared. The preacher must absorb the sermon within his or her own heart. Whether or not one preaches from manuscript, outline, or extemporaneously, the message should be apart of the preacher. Dr. Terry Thomas says, "I have my sermon written out, but I have to internalize my sermon. The sermon has to be alive in my heart and active in my memory."[101] The psalmist has declared, "Your word I have treasured in my heart."[102] Many homiletics instructors have suggested a daily pattern during the week for sermonic preparation, such as the late Dr. Samuel DeWitt Proctor's *The Certain Sound of the Trumpet* and Calvin Miller's *Marketplace Preaching* to name a few.

The work of the preacher on Monday involves the selection of the given biblical text, title and focus of the sermon, and the forming of the proposition or thesis. The late Dr. Miles J. Jones identified this initial act of preparation as the "organizing observation." "The organizing observation can be brought about by the rendering of two basic questions: What is the condition of existence made evident by this text? In what ways does this text address that condition?"[103] Monday's work will also involve the act of "free association" within the biblical text as suggested by Dr. Frank A. Thomas. "the methodology for free association is to write either the biblical text or the sermon idea in the

---

101 Dr. Terry Thomas, "From Hunch to Proclamation"
102 Ps. 119:11 (NAS)
103 Dr. Miles J. Jones, "Introductory Homiletics", (notes from lecture delivered at the Samuel DeWitt Proctor School of Theology at Virginia Union University, Richmond, VA).

center of a blank sheet of paper and allow whatever thoughts, feelings, images, or ideas that come to mind to be recorded."[104]

Tuesday is the day of consulting commentaries and doing word studies in the original languages of the given biblical text. The danger of consulting commentaries on Monday may result in thwarting the connection and direction that the Holy Spirit may intend for the sermon However, Tuesday's work also includes consulting other biblical translations for relevancy. "Greek and Hebrew word studies often prepackage simple, hurried words as metaphors of power. These classic metaphors will link with contemporary illustrations to freshen and vitalize dull sermons. Eugene Peterson's new work, *The Message*, is a must. Peterson's grasp of synonyms and the richness of the English language fill the text with light."[105]

Wednesday is the day of developing an introduction, choosing illustrations, or selecting appropriate statistics and poetry as needed to contemporize biblical ideas. In order to develop a relevant word for this 21st century people, the scriptural ideas need to be relational to the substance of what people are faced with in today's world. Dr. Terry Thomas notes:

> To make the connection between my world and the world in which the text was written, I have to draw an analogy. To draw an analogy is to make a comparison between the similar features or attributes of two otherwise dissimilar things, so that the unknown, or less well known, is clarified by the known. The use of analogy means a grasping of patterns of similarity between the scripture and the Christian experience today. It is an act of imagination.[106]

---

104 Frank A. Thomas, *They Liked to Never Quit Praisin' God*, 66.
105 Calvin Miller, *Marketplace Preaching: How to Return the Sermon to Where it Belongs*, 152-153.
106 Dr. Terry Thomas, "From Hunch to Proclamation"

Thursday is the day of actually crafting the sermon. It is always a good idea, for clarity purposes, for one to completely write out the sermon in manuscript form. Regardless of delivery preferences, manuscript, outline, or extemporaneously, writing out the sermon helps to solidify the essence of what the preacher is attempting to say to the people within the pews. "If the sermon is perfectly crafted, it will not wander off aimlessly toward an indefinable conclusion. If the conclusion is crafted very carefully, both the preacher and the congregation will realize when the sermon is finished."[107] Crafting the message from start to finish will have a great impact upon the preacher and the pew. The second habit of Stephen R. Covey's *The Seven Habits of Highly Effective People*, is to begin with the end in mind. "To begin with the end in mind means to start with a clear understanding of your destination. It means to know where you're going so that you better understand where you are now and so that the steps you take are always in the right direction."[108] "The importance of the closing stage of celebration to African American preaching is witnessed in the fact that the luminary preacher Martin Luther King, Jr., in a conversation about the first steps of sermon preparation, said, 'The first thing I think about is how I am going to close.'"[109] According to Wyatt T. Walker, the first thing King considered in preparation was the strategy for celebration."[110]

Friday and early Saturday morning are days of "polishing" the sermon with the necessary transitions, moves, and structures as

---

107 Calvin Miller, *Marketplace Preaching: How to Return the Sermon to Where It Belongs*, 159.

108 Stephen R. Covey, *The Seven Habits of Highly Effective People: Powerful Lessons in Personal Change*, (New York: Fireside Simon & Shuster, 1989), 98.

109 Wyatt T. Walker, *The Soul of Black Worship*, (New York: Martin Luther King Fellows Press, 1984), 17.

110 Frank A. Thomas, *They Liked to Never Quit Praisin' God*, 77.

noted by David Buttrick's *Homiletic Moves and Structures*.[111] This phase of preparation is vital, if the sermon is going to be effective. The sermon should have transitions to connect the major points of the message and to "guard against stagnation and backwash."[112] The moves and structures of the message should be strategic and brief, remembering that 21st century people are somewhat impatient and the preacher needs to get to the point efficiently. "The average Westerner now has no more than a three-minute attention span. It is important that the movements, therefore, do not take more time than the average attention span allows."[113]

Finally, when the sermon has been polished and the outline or thought internalized, the preacher must be well-rested for the preaching moment. How can one deliver a word that is fresh and relevant in this 21st century, if he or she is tired, weary, and worn? Dr. Ricky Woods says, "Something goes lacking whenever we bring tired bodies to the pulpit. Much of what the preacher does can be done by someone else but he preacher must preach. Therefore, come each week to the pulpit with a rested body and ready to preach. Some practical suggestions on how to maintain a rested body for Sunday morning includes the following: limit weekend activities beginning Friday evening, maintain a proper and healthy diet with exercise, plan time for leisure each week, and go to bed early Saturday night."[114] The task of preaching with relevancy requires much preparation, but after the benediction has been given, it shall be worth it all.

---

111 David G. Buttrick, *Homiletic Moves and Structures*, (Philadelphia: Fortress Press, 1987).
112 Calvin Miller, *Marketplace Preaching: How to Return the Sermon to Where it Belongs*, 163.
113 Ibid, 164.
114 Dr. Ricky Woods, "Getting Ready to Preach"

Theoretical Foundation

THE FOCAL POINT OF CHAPTER three is to establish a theoretical foundation for equipping and empowering rural church leaders in 21st century ministry through health awareness. The historical, biblical, and theological components discussed here will provide a structure upon which the ministry model will be developed and implemented. Although the theoretical foundations will establish a framework, the process through which the level of health awareness will be raised is through preaching.

Theological Foundations

The guiding theological premise of this ministry project is primarily grounded in components of practical theology. It is the premise of the writer that God is much concerned about the health and welfare of humanity, particularly those in need. Isaiah 58: 6-8 states:

> Is not this the fast that I have chosen? To loose the bands of wickedness, to undo the heavy burdens, and

> to let the oppressed go free, and that ye break every
> yoke? Is it not to deal thy bread to the hungry, and
> that thou bring the poor that are cast out to thy house?
> When thou seest the naked, that thou cover him; and
> that thou hide not thyself from thine own flesh? Then
> shall thy light break forth as the morning, and thine
> health shall spring forth speedily; and thy righteous-
> ness shall go before thee; the glory of the Lord shall
> be thy rereward.

God's concern for the welfare and well-being of humankind can also
be supported by John 3:17 "For God sent not his Son into the world to
condemn the world; but that the world through him might be saved."
Furthermore, this concern is made evident through the preaching
and reaching ministry of Christ. For instance in Luke 7:22 and Luke
14:12-14, respectively:

> Then Jesus answering said unto them, Go your way,
> and tell John what things ye have seen and heard;
> how that the blind see, the lame walk, the lepers are
> cleansed, the deaf hear, the dead are raised, to the
> poor the gospel is preached.

> Then said he also to him that bade him, When thou
> makest a dinner of a supper, call not thy friends, nor
> thy brethren, neither thy kinsmen, nor thy rich neigh-
> bors; lest they also bid thee again, and a recompense
> be made thee. But when thou makest a feast, call the
> poor, the maimed, the lame, the blind: and thou shalt
> be blessed...

The very foundation of Jesus' earthly ministry was holistic healing
and health awareness through practical application, particularly to
those in great need. Dr. James H. Harris holds that:

The message of Jesus is one that is addressed to the despised and oppressed. He comforts and strengthens the weak, feeds the hungry, and heals the sick of their diseases—those who are on the "underside of culture.[115]

"At the synagogue, Jesus explained his mission as one of bringing good news to the poor and the suffering (Luke 4). He also says, "Come to me, all you who are weary and burdened, and I will give you rest (Matt. 11:28)."[116]

Although a great many people assume that the Bible is strictly a religious book dealing exclusively with "spiritual" matters, even a casual study of the Scriptures reveals that they deal with [humanity] as a whole person—body, mind, and spirit. The biblical text is largely directed to nurturing, protecting, and guiding human beings to achieve their full potential in every area of their being.[117]

This is what Jesus meant in John 10:10b when he stated: "...I am come that they might have life, and that they might have it more abundantly." It is the objective of the writer to carefully point out the component factors which ground this ministry project through a practical theology of "preaching" and "reaching" for the purpose of health awareness in the rural context.

Olin P. Moyd offers a working definition of "practical theology" stating that:

---

115 James H. Harris, *Pastoral Theology: A Black Church Perspective*, (Minneapolis: Fortress Press, 1991), 24.

116 John Perkins, *Beyond Charity: The Call To Christian Community Development*, (Grand Rapids: Baker Books, 1993) 45.

117 Reginald Cherry, M.D., *Healing Prayer: God's Divine Intervention in Medicine, Faith, and Prayer*, (Nashville: Thomas Nelson Publishers, 1999) 46.

> Practical theology reflects upon the divine mandate
> for ministries through the church. It examines both
> the biblical mandate and the present human condi-
> tion and attempts to correlate the two, giving divine
> sanction to the mission and ministries of the church
> in every current world situation.[118]

The field of practical theology has historically been subdivided into the following disciplines: pastoral care, homiletics, Christian Education, liturgics, social services, congregational studies, and church development. Practical theology is the integration of theology and the various facets of ministry as they relate to the church and society as a whole. In light of the fact that Andrew Purves asserts that "practical theology is concerned with action" it is the contention of the writer that practical theology focuses more towards the "hands-on" approach.

Health awareness ministry is an application of the "hands-on" approach. There are at least three instances in Luke the physician's Gospel account of Jesus utilizing the "hands-on" approach to ministry for the promotion of health and wellness. In Luke 5:24-25, Jesus speaks a word of empowerment to a man "sick of the palsy" to "arise, and take up thy couch, and go into thine house." In Luke 6:8-10, Jesus again speaks a word of empowerment to a man whose right hand was withered saying, "rise up, and stand forth in the midst." In Luke 13:11-13, Jesus speaks a word of empowerment and lays hands on a woman which had been sick and bent over for eighteen years saying:

> Woman, thou are loosed from thine infirmity. And he
> laid his hands on her: and immediately she was made
> straight, and glorified God.

---

118 Olin P. Moyd, *The Sacred Art: Preaching and Theology in the African American Tradition*, (Valley Forge: Judson Press, 1995) 34.

Friedrich Daniel Ernst Schleiermacher, renowned theologian and philosopher is credited by many scholars as the "father of practical theology." Schleiermacher was born on November 21, 1768 in Breslau and was the son of a Prussian army chaplain of the Reformed confession.[119] Paul Tillich asserts:

> Friedreich Schleiermacher praised practical theology as the crown of theology. For Schleiermacher, practical theology was not a third part of theology in addition to historical and systematic theology but rather the technical theory through which the other two parts, the historical and the systematic, were to be applied in the life of the church.[120]

Schleiermacher was able to make a significant contribution to the field of practical theology because of the fact that he was not only a scholar in the academy, but he was able to gather experience in the disciplines of preaching and teaching.

> While he preached every Sunday, he also gradually took up his lectures in the university in almost every branch of theology and philosophy—New Testament exegesis, introduction to and interpretation of the New Testament, ethics (both philosophic and Christian), dogmatic and practical theology, church history, history of philosophy, psychology, dialectics (logic and metaphysics), politics, pedagogy, translation and aesthetics....*as a preacher he produced a powerful effect, yet not at all by the force of his oratory but by his intellectual strength, his devotional spirit and the philosophical breadth and unity of his thought.*"[121]

---

119 http://en.wikipedia.org/wiki/Friedrich_Schleiermacher
120 Paul Tillich, *Systematic Theology, Book I,* (Chicago: University of Chicago Press, 1971) 32.
121 http://en.wikipedia.org/wiki/Friedrich_Schleiermacher (emphasis added)

The preaching and teaching ministry has often served as the model by which individuals have become persuaded, informed, empowered, and equipped for action or attitudinal change. "One of the most important elements in the preaching event was persuasion."[122] Therefore, it is the intent of the writer to define a theology of preaching, particularly in light of a health awareness ministry model within a rural context.

A Theology of Preaching

The time has come for the Christian church to rise to the occasion and bring forth the Gospel of Jesus Christ like never before to a generation that is in desperate and dire need of relevant preachment. According to Jerry Vines and Jim Shaddix in their work entitled, *Power in the Pulpit*, "Preaching…is informed by the biblical emphasis on the practical application of God's Word to the lives of contemporary listeners."[123] Although this world is in a constant state of change, there is however, one thing that remains the same, that is the Gospel or the "Good News" of Jesus the Christ and the Great Commission that has been given to the church to "Go into all the world and preach the gospel to all creation."[124] It appears as if there has never been a time when the needs of so many have been so great. With the advent of this new millennium, one can clearly see that the increase of religious, ethical, and cultural pluralism accelerated by rapid technological change is drastically affecting the fabric of our economy and society. The end result often leads to a climate of increasing uncertainty, chaos, and confusion. Gospel preachers across the length and breadth

---

122 Jerry Vines and Jim Shaddix, *Power in the Pulpit: How to Prepare and Deliver Expository Sermons*, (Chicago: Moody Press, 1999), 23.
123 Ibid, 20.
124 Mk. 16:15 New American Standard Bible

of America and the world for that matter, have an awesome task to bring forth a "Word" that is both, practical and relevant in this 21st Century, particularly in the area of health and wellness. The definition of relevant includes "having significant and demonstrable bearing on the matter at hand; practical and especially social applicability."[125] This is exactly what Jesus did throughout the three and one-half years of his earthly ministry, particularly for the sick, suffering, and those in need of an empowering word for health, healing, and a new start. Gospel preachers are challenged to re-examine their role and effectiveness in light of contemporary society and to take the positive steps towards becoming more relevant within the church and throughout the world. Professor Melva Wilson Costen states that:

> While currently a variety of preaching styles is utilized in Black worship, the traditional perception is that the preacher is able to "tell the story" (literally communicate) in language, symbols, and symbolic mannerisms that speak directly to the needs of worshipers.[126]

There is a great need for preaching that will address the matters at hand as well as the vicissitudes of life, both significantly and practically. It is the aim of this ministry model of health awareness to inform, inspire, and influence people through practical preaching to deal with the issue of being holy and whole. One of the underlying theological principles of this health awareness ministry model is that preaching with relevancy and effectiveness will require the preacher to focus not just on the salvific acts of God, but how God is concerned about the total person. Cleophus J. LaRue asserts:

---

125 *Merriam-Webster's Collegiate Dictionary*, 10th Edition (1999: Philippines), 987.

126 Melva Wilson Costen, *African American Christian Worship*,,(Nashville: Abingdon Press, 1993), 105.

> The most effective preaching is preaching that conveys with clarity and insight how God acts in concrete situations in the lives of those who hear the gospel. People gather to be assured and reassured that God has acted and will act for them and for their salvation.[127]

The work of the preacher is clearly "cut out" for him or her, particularly in this 21st Century. The issue of clarity, effectiveness, and relevance for today's world within the preachment is paramount. The Apostle Paul challenged and charged Timothy, his son in the Gospel ministry to, "Preach the word; be ready in season and out of season."[128] The responsibility of the preacher is to preach God's word even in the midst of "season transitions."

> The preacher is compelled to say something that addresses the needs of the people, directing the message to their heart and head. The sermon needs to be powerful enough to motivate churchgoers to live a life that reflects the spirit of Jesus Christ.[129]

Now, to live a life that mirrors the spirit of Jesus Christ is to live a life that exhibits concern for the physical, mental, and spiritual health and well-being of self as well as in others which is an example of "health awareness in action." Did not Jesus once say in Matthew 25:42-43:

> For I was an hungred, and ye gave me no meat: I was thirsty, and ye gave me no drink: I was a stranger, and ye took me not in: naked, and ye clothed me not: sick, and in prison, and ye visited me not.

---

127 Cleophus J. Larue, *The Heart of Black Preaching*, (Louisville, Kentucky: Westminster John Knox Press, 2000), 69.

128 II Tim. 4:2 (New American Standard)

129 James H. Harris, *Pastoral Theology: A Black Church Perspective*, (Minneapolis: Fortress Press, 1991), 98-99.

This issue of relevancy for this present season may require the initiation of a discussion or dialogue on the way we do practical theology and the study of preaching as a whole. If there is no discourse in this regard, there is a risk that the church will become irrelevant at precisely the time when its hour has come. Gospel preaching in this 21st Century that is relevant, effective, and applicable will require the preacher to preach with a powerful effect.

Preaching a relevant word in this 21st century requires power. The working definition of power for this discourse is "the ability to act or produce an effect."[130] Gospel preaching in this new millennium must have an effect or produce results in the lives of the hearers. In order to be effective, preachers must return to the biblical foundations upon which the craft of preaching rests: the apostolic and early church forerunners. The preaching of the Christian message was primarily given birth under intense persecution and tribulation as recorded within the Acts of the Apostles and throughout the New Testament. Even in the midst of a time period when preaching the good news of Christ was not popular at all, the Apostle Paul declares, "I am not ashamed of the gospel, for it is the power of God for salvation to everyone who believes, to the Jew first and also to the Greek."[131] Frank A. Thomas states:

> Preaching is a spiritual gift given by the Holy Spirit to help the church and the world receive and celebrate the good news of Christ. Through the spiritual gift of preaching, people are led to an experience of the assurance of grace, and the church fulfills its mission to proclaim the good news to the world."[132]

130 *Merriam-Webster's Collegiate Dictionary*, 10th ed., (Springfield, Mass. 1999), 913.
131 Rom. 1:16 New American Standard
132 Frank A. Thomas, *They Like to Never Quit Praisin' God: The Role of Celebration in Preaching*, (Cleveland: United Church Press, 1997), 27.

During these times, the preacher of the Gospel ought to have fervor and fire when preaching this liberating Message. The preaching moment is no time to be doubtful, timid, and ashamed. In order to preach with power, one must have a clear understanding of this glorious gospel that they are preaching.

What is preaching the gospel all about? According to the late Miles J. Jones:

> Christian preaching is all about Jesus Christ. Every sermon preached is to be informed by a kerygmatic content. Preaching in the early church was based on the "kerygma", which consists of the life, death, resurrection, and an urge to respond to Christ. Kerygma is the essential and distinguishing ingredient of Christian preaching and the interpretive key to our ethnic particularity.[133]

In order to preach a relevant word with power to produce an effect in the lives of the hearers, the focus must be upon the risen Christ. Dr. James H. Harris argues:

> In order to preach the gospel, the preacher needs to have a clear understanding of Christology, that is, probing the nature and meaning of Jesus for the church today. For the Christian, faith in Jesus Christ as redeemer and savior is the glue that holds the church together as a community of believers. In a time of troubling apathy, coupled with spiritual and social malaise in the church and society, the meaning of Jesus Christ gains new relevance.[134]

---

133 Dr. Miles J. Jones, (lecture presented at the Samuel Dewitt Proctor School of Theology, Richmond, Virginia, December 1997).

134 James H. Harris, *Preaching Liberation*, (Minneapolis: Fortress Press, 1995), 27.

True gospel preaching that is practical, powerful, and applicable will provoke transformation and change for the betterment of humanity in a manner that is holistic. In Acts 2:14-36, after the Apostle Peter proclaimed the Gospel message with boldness and power, the hearers "were pricked in their heart and said to Peter and the rest of the apostles, Men and brethren, 'what shall we do?'" It is the contention of the writer, that many individuals will not change lifestyle habits that lead to negative and unhealthy outcomes until they are "pricked in their heart" and confronted with the whole Gospel of Jesus Christ. It is only when the preacher deliberately and purposely sets out to inform, inspire, and educate the congregants about living a healthy and holistic lifestyle through the power of the Biblical text, that individuals will begin to ask the question, "What shall we do?" Carlyle Fielding Steward III also contends that:

> Proclamation is the process of announcing something. In the case of Christianity, the church proclaims the Good News of the Risen Christ, one who vanquishes evil and death through the resurrection. This victorious attitude is bequeathed to those who possess and profess faith in him, and it is open to those who freely and joyfully follow him. But more than lip service, it requires principles and action-oriented behavior.[135]

Theology of Reaching

Preaching a relevant word with power can be very liberating. The earthly preaching, teaching, and reaching ministry of Jesus was one of deliverance. It was practical and relevant. The ministry of Jesus produced change, transformation, and evoked a response. Jesus

---

135 Carlyle Fielding Stewart III, *African American Church Growth: 12 Principles for Prophetic Ministry*, (Nashville: Abingdon Press, 1994), 116.

asserted that his very presence and ministry on the earth was in fulfillment of the prophecy in the sixty-first chapter of Isaiah:

> The Spirit of the Lord is upon me, because He anointed me to preach the Gospel to the poor, He as sent me to proclaim release to the captives, and recovery of sight to the blind, to set free those who are oppressed, to proclaim the favorable year of the Lord. And he closed the book, gave it back to the attendant and sat down: and the eyes of all the synagogue were fixed on Him. And he began to say to them, Today this Scripture has been fulfilled in your hearing.[136]

This good news that Christ has come and will come again is liberating particularly to those within the African-American faith community. Dr. Frank A. Thomas says:

> The nature and purpose of African-American preaching is to help people experience the assurance of grace (good news) that is the gospel of Jesus the Christ. It is this assurance of grace, received through African American preaching and worship that has historically sustained, encouraged, and liberated African American people.[137]

Effective gospel preaching that is truly packed with power ought to liberate and set people free, physically, mentally, and spiritually. Carlyle Fielding Steward III states:

> We say that the preached word is an important element of evangelism because in the Protestant tradition the kerygma is an indispensable part of worship. Black people as a rule will attend a church where

---

136 Lk. 4:18-21 New American Standard
137 Frank A. Thomas, *They Like to Never Quit Praisin' God: The Role of Celebration in Preaching*, (Cleveland: United Church Press, 1997), 3.

there's good preaching, but more important, it must be preaching that faithfully proclaims the tenets of a crucified, resurrected, and liberating Christ![138]

In order for gospel preaching to be powerful and effective, the preacher must identify and address needs of the hearers in a way that is practical and understandable. It has been said often that "if it doesn't make sense to the preacher, then it probably won't be clear to those within the pews." If people in the pews are going to be set free by the power of God, it is absolutely necessary for the preacher to "make it plain." Dr. Frank A. Thomas contends "people rarely experience the sermon if the preacher does not experience it first."[139] It may be necessary for preachers to begin preaching messages on Sunday that are more practical versus the theoretical sermon. Charles Jefferson speaks to this issue:

> There are two kinds of preaching. There is what we may call "Academic" preaching, the unfolding of ideas and truths for the sake of the ideas and truths themselves....It is always interesting work o take an idea or principle and give an exposition of it, unfolding its beauty, exploring its meaning. Many rejoice in that sort of intellectual work, and many other people greatly enjoy seeing them do it....On the other hand is "Practical" preaching...I am not interested in abstractions in the pulpit. In my library at home, with books of philosophy around me, I can have a good time in the realm of theory and speculation, but as soon as I get into the pulpit, I am always practical...I care noth-

---

138 Carlyle Fielding Stewart III, *African American Church Growth: 12 Principles for Prophetic Ministry*, 122.

139 Frank A. Thomas, *They Like to Never Quit Praisin' God: The Role of Celebration in Preaching*, 37.

ing for the unfolding of ideas unless I can apply them
to the conduct of individuals and institutions.[140]

Preaching and teaching for the purpose of health awareness in the
local church may require a more practical methodology for sermon
preparation and delivery in order to be effective. Cleophus J. LaRue,
the Francis Landey Patton Associate Professor of Homiletics at
Princeton Theological Seminary asserts:

> Understanding the multifaceted life situations of
> blacks is important to the crafting of the sermon be-
> cause of the manner in which black listeners process
> the gospel. Blacks are more inclined to hear the gospel
> through life experiences rather than through codified
> theological formulations.[141]

Dr. Terry Thomas, pastor of the West Durham Baptist Church,
provides an excellent example of preaching the gospel through life
experience in a sermon on health awareness entitled: "Maintaining
your health while going through the storm" based on Acts 27:33-37.
Dr. Thomas states, "Listen, a storm may not directly touch you, but
if the storm can cause you to do hard or neglect your health, the
storm has found an inroad to obtain the victory over your life."[142]
Many parishioners bring their burdens with them to church. They
turn to the church week after week for spiritual solace and sanctuary
from a sinful world. The burning question in the hearts and minds
of many is interrogated as such: "Is there a word from the Lord, for
my situation in life?" James Earl Massey states:

---

140 Jay E. Adams, *Truth Applied*, (Grand Rapids: Zondervan Publishing, 1990),
      33-34.
141 Cleophus J. LaRue, *The Heart of Black Preaching*, 123.
142 Dr. Terry Thomas in a sermon preached at West Durham Baptist Church,
      Durham Baptist Church (unpublished material).

To preach black, then, is to preach out of an awareness of the issues and concerns of life with which blacks struggle and contend with daily. The black sermon at its best arises out of the totality of the people's existence—their pain, joy, trouble, and ecstasy.[143]

Liberation in the pews can only take place if and when the preacher begins to address the "everyday" issues of life that people are constantly faced with. Health awareness is one of those "everyday" issues that has a lasting effect upon people's lives that needs to be addressed practically from the pulpit. Dr. James H. Harris, pastor of the Second Baptist Church of Richmond, Virginia states:

Today, in addition to theological training, the black preacher needs to understand economics, history, and political theory in order to address the many needs of the black church. The context of black preaching is one of urban and rural poverty, joblessness, homelessness, discrimination, and to a lesser degree, black individual success, educational achievement, and economic independence.[144]

Furthermore, the message of Jesus Christ can be liberating and effective when the preacher surrenders his or her gifts to the Eternal One to be used at that sacred moment for the needs of the hearers. The preacher must become informed, through reading, observation, and relationship, with the heartbeat of the congregation so that God's word will flow freely and produce much fruit in the lives of the parishioners. "Melva W. Costen contends that:

---

143 James Earl Massey, *The Responsible Pulpit*, (Anderson, Indiana: Warner Press, 1974), 101-10.
144 James H. Harris, *Preaching Liberation*, 51.

> The messenger brings to the task a variety of gifts: knowledge of the word, a divine listening ear, and a "feel" for the gathered community. With these gifts, the preacher serves as a divine conduit through which the fresh Word of God can flow without encumbrance.[145]

Liberation within the preachment comes as a result of the preacher's God-given ability to simply "tell the story" in such a way that it becomes just as fresh and relevant as the day it actually happened. Costen further argues that:

> An important characteristic of hermeneutics in Black preaching is the empowerment of the preacher to create an atmosphere wherein the preacher and listener might hear the Word by experiencing it. The preacher must be so familiar with the story that he or she, during the preaching moment, becomes the biblical character, the carrier of the letter from the epistle writer to the people, the paralytic who needs healing, or the woman with the issue of blood. The *sitz in leben* ("situation in life") of the text is internalized so that it is transformed, and it comes alive to the context of the preacher. The goal is to create an atmosphere in which the listeners can themselves become the word of God incarnate at the moment."[146]

This "theology of reaching" not only encompasses the preaching ministry of Christ, but the compassion of Christ as well. According to Matthew 14:14, Mark 6:34, and Mark 8:1-2, Jesus didn't just come preaching a word, but Jesus came with great compassion and concern for the people. "The entire life and ministry of Jesus demonstrates of Jesus' concern for persons in their human hurts, as well as His

---

145 Melva Wilson Costen, *African American Christian Worship*, 105.
146 Ibid, 130-131.

concern for people finding salvation through a personal relationship with God."[147] The theological foundation of this ministry projects rests in the need to emulate the ministry of Christ through the health and healing of those in need.

> In carrying out his ministry, Jesus seemingly operated under the influence of his compassion. Jesus' compassion appeared to be the prompter that motivated him to meet the needs of people. It was that which was intrinsic about Jesus that seemingly motivated Jesus to respond affirmatively and responsibly to people whose situation prevented them from advancing in life holistically or threatened their well being.[148]

Historical Foundations for the Ministry Focus

The historical foundation of this project is firmly rooted and grounded in the fact that many African-Americans, particularly those within the rural context of ministry, have made choices that have had a negative impact upon their health conditions throughout the years. The need for more health awareness ministry models within the African-American rural church context is imperative, due to the fact that studies have repeatedly proven that many African-Americans in these areas have been subject to poor health conditions and outcomes. Furthermore, the lack of knowledge as it pertains to eating a healthy diet has historically had a significant affect upon the rural African-American community which can be traced back to American slavery. August Meier and Elliott Rudwick in their book

---

147 Findley B. Edge, *The Doctrine of the Laity*, (Nashville: Convention Press, 1985), 62.

148 Dr. Terry Thomas, "Compassionate Christ and Church", (lecture notes taken from UTS Peer Session at Orlando, Florida) unpublished material.

entitled, *From Plantation to Ghetto*, speak of the unhealthy slave conditions stating:

> ...most slaves lived in rude, drafty, leaky, clapboard shacks, with only the crudest furniture. As for clothing, a standard winter supply for a man was two shirts of coarse cotton, two woolen trousers, and a woolen jacket. Every year he received a pair of shoes. The standard food allowance consisted of hominy and fatback, with a basic weekly ration of a peck of cornmeal and three or four pounds of salt pork.[149]

According to Healthy People 2010, African-Americans account for only 12% of the population in the United States, yet African-Americans, as a group, have the poorest health status indicators in the nation and are disproportionately represented among underserved populations."[150] There is a tremendous need for health awareness through preaching within the African-American rural communities, because many African-Americans continue to make bad choices that often lead to disease and infirmity.

> African-Americans continue to be two times more likely than whites to have hypertension, obesity, and high fat intake. Poor nutrition, smoking, alcohol, and drug abuse are reported to occur commonly in African-American women thereby increasing the risk for heart disease and type two diabetes.[151]

---

149 August Meier and Elliott Rudwick, *From Plantation to Ghetto*, (New York: Hill and Wang, 1976), 67.

150 U.S. Department of Health and Human Services. *Developing objectives for health people 2010*. Washington, D.C.: Government Printing Office, 2002.

151 C.M. Davis and C.M. Curley, "Disparities of health in African-Americans," *Nursing Clinics of North America* (1999): 34,345-357.

"The lack of access to preventative care, a stressful lifestyle, poor education, inadequate housing, low paying jobs, and a lack of insurance are powerful predictors of health outcomes."[152] "Healthy People 2010 statistics indicate that African-Americans do not consistently receive enough early, routine, and preventative healthcare."[153] "The major health disparities among many racially and ethnically diverse people with low income is ample evidence of lack of access to health care and an ongoing dire need for improved health access and health promotion in those communities."[154] These historical findings traced from American slavery to the present-time further substantiate the need for a health awareness ministry model through preaching in the rural context. One of the things that preaching does is inform. Holistic ministry is about informing that which is essential to an abundant life.

The health concerns in the rural context differ from the urban setting and much awareness is needed. "Rural America finds itself caught in an ever-deepening health care crisis."[155]

> The closing of light industry and family businesses causes young people to migrate to cities and suburbs. Because those who remain tend to be elderly and unemployed and/or uninsured, they further strain the resources of already—struggling rural hospitals and clinics. Meanwhile, the financial difficulties faced

---

152 E.J. Bailey, "Sociocultural factors and health care-seeking behavior among Black Americnas," *Journal of the National Medical Association* (1987): 79, 389-392.

153 U.S. Department of Health and Human Services, *Health Status of minorities and low income groups*. Washington, D.C.: U.S. Government Printing Office, (1991).

154 S. Drayton-Hargrove and J.H. Woods, "Ethical analysis of health care reform: Implications for diverse communities," *The ABNF Journal* (1995): 6, 99-103.

155 "A special eight-article section on the crisis and responses by Catholic health care organizations toit," *Health Progress* (March/April 2004): 14-35,50-53.

by these hospitals and clinics tend to make them unattractive to physicians, nurses, and other medical professionals. As a result, rural people receive less and less care.[156]

According to Shannon Jung, director of the Center for Theology and Land, an outreach ministry of the University of Dubuque and Wartburg theological seminaries:

> Some rural communities have ceased to be the center of services for their counties. Neither do towns and localities serve as profit centers for their counties but have instead become profit centers for others...At present, however, these communities have lost hospitals and immediate access to medical services.[157]

The connection between rural health and economics can be viewed by many as a sad commentary, because "poverty among rural families and rural communities is increasing."[158] According to John M. Perkins, founder of Voice of Calvary Ministries in Jackson, Mississippi,

> The link between poverty and health is simple. First, the poor rarely have the knowledge or resources common to middle-class America for preventive care, such as a healthy diet and simple lifestyle measures that can lead to a healthier body...When emergencies occur, the poor cannot afford to pay for essential services, and over a lifetime, debilitating conditions can result. While a well-employed middle-class citizen produces an insurance card at a suburban hospital and receives care, the inner-city emergency room closes down due

---

156 Margot K. Hover, "Rural clergy and Holistic Care," *Health Progress* (September/October 2005).

157 Shannon Jung, *Rural Ministry: The Shape of the Renewal to Come* (Nashville: Abingdon Press, 1998), 111-112.

158 Ibid, 113.

to lack of funds and the poor are often refused any but the bare minimum of treatment without insurance.[159]

It is within these despairing conditions that African-American church must rise up and rededicate itself to its historical role within the rural community.

Historically, the African-American church has always been the "haven" or "hub" of services, addressing both the spiritual and physical needs within the community.

> Although not particularly visible in the formal rural church movement—given the constraints of legal and cultural segregation—the black churches were significant institutions in the lives of rural blacks, most of whom resided in southern states. The churches functioned as the most significant cultural institutions, the locations for black self-expression, and the sources of leadership for the black community. Churches organized many of the services denied or limited to blacks under racists governments in the southern states—including high schools and healthcare.[160]

According to W.E.B. DuBois, author of the *Souls of Black Folk*, "A people must have a social center and that center for African-Americans has traditionally been the church. Since emancipation, the African-American church has become more organized as a government with a head who can influence every aspect of life."[161] Rural church leaders must reclaim their prophetic leadership responsibility within the community, particularly as it relates to health awareness.

---

159 John M. Perkins, *Beyond Charity: The Call to Christian Community Development* (Grand Rapids, MI: Baker Books, 1993), 98-99.

160 Shannon Jung, *Rural Ministry: The Shape of the Renewal to Come* (Nashville, TN: Abingdon Press, 1998), 45-46.

161 W.E.B. DuBois, *The Souls of Black Folk* (New York: Vintage Books, 1903).

> The pastor in the African-American church is a healer of the sick, an interpreter of the unknown, and comforter for the sorrowed. Church nurse units, church nurse guilds, and healthcare ministries have historically provided a trusted social network for health education, encouragement, and support.[162]

"If health status indicators are to improve for African-American populations, then new culturally relevant, credible, and trusted approaches to providing healthcare services must be identified."[163] There is a vital need for the local church to return to its heritage and provide meaningful ministry that touches the mind, body, and soul. This project calls for a radical reversal of the church's role. It is imperative that the church not only address issues of morality, but must address those physical issues as well.

> It is practically impossible to do effective holistic ministry apart from the local church. A nurturing community of faith can best provide the thrusts of evangelism, discipleship, spiritual accountability and relationship by which disciples grow in their walk with God.[164]

"Although churches are not traditional health care settings based on the standards of modern medicine, faith communities have been actively involved in providing health care for centuries."[165]

---

162 V.J. Briscoe and J.W. Pichert, "Promoting utilization of health care services through the African-American church," *The ABNF Journal* (1997): 7.

163 Ibid, 129-132.

164 John M. Perkins, *Restoring At-Risk Communities: Doing It Together and Doing It Right* (Grand Rapids, MI: Baker Books, 1995), 23.

165 M.J. Schank, D. Weiss, and R. Mathevs, "Parish nursing: ministry of healing," *Geriatric Nursing* (1996), 17, 1-3.

Studies have repeatedly exhibited the powerful and positive impact of the local church's involvement in the lives of its members and adherents as it relates to improved health outcomes.

> People who practice their religious faith regularly may be getting some earthly benefits: they appear to be healthier compared to people who never attend a house of worship. A study conducted by sociologists at Perdue University in West Lafayette, Indiana, found that 4% of those who regularly went to church or synagogue reported poor health, compared with 9% of those who did not attend a house of worship. And 36% of weekly worshippers reported they were in excellent health, compared with 26% of non-attenders. Why the difference? Researchers aren't sure, but they say the reason may be that people attending weekly services may be more likely to see friends who ask about their health and can recommend a doctor.[166]

The writer shall cite four recent studies conducted in the realm of health awareness in conjunction with the church.

> Research has shown that church parishes can play a pivotal role in their parishioners' health. In one study, a group of people with musculoskeletal disabilities was asked how they were able to continue to perform their normal activities despite those problems; all credited their spiritual lives with giving them needed strength and resilience.[167]

> Another study involved rural breast cancer survivors who were trained to protect themselves from recurrence of the illness through self-examination and

---

166 *Spokesman Review,* (October 1992).
167 K. Faull, M. Hills, G. Cochrane, et al., "Investigation of Health Perspectives of Those with Physical Disabilities: The Role of Spirituality as a Determinant of Health," *Disability Rehabilitation* 26, no. 3 (2004): 129-144.

mammography. The training resulted in significantly increased screening activity in the study area, and this success was partly attributed to the fact that the program was based in and encouraged by the church to which many of the participants belonged.[168]

A third study explored the meaning that a group of rural people attached to certain unconventional remedies for arthritis. The researchers found that while members of the group were generally skeptical about the remedies' effectiveness, the language they used was heavily freighted with such terms as "faith", "transformation", "communion", "self-help", and "spiritual healing".[169] "The study suggested that religion and religious ideas remain important in rural America, and because they do, can themselves have a therapeutic effect in the treatment of rural people."[170]

Furthermore, a successful study was conducted among fifty African-American congregations in ten different rural counties throughout the state of North Carolina in collaboration with the National Cancer Institute (NCI).

This study assessed the effects of the Black Churches United for Better Health project on increasing fruit and vegetable consumption among rural African American church members in North Carolina. Ten counties comprising 50 churches were pair matched and

---

168 D.O. Erwin, T.S. Spatz, R.C. Stotts, et al., "Increasing Mammography Practice among African-American Women," *Cancer Practice* 7, no. 2 (February 1999): 78-85.

169 T.A. Arcury, W.M. Gesier, and H.L. Cook, "Meaning in the Use of Unconventional Arthritis Therapies," *American Journal of Health Promotion* 14, no. 1 (September/October 1999): 7-15.

170 Margot K. Hover, "Rural Clergy and Holistic Care," *Health Progress* (September/October 2005).

randomly assigned to either intervention or delayed intervention conditions. A multicomponent intervention was conducted over approximately 20 months. A total of 2519 adults (77.3% response rate) completed both the baseline and 2-year follow-up interviews. The 2 study groups consumed similar amounts of fruits and vegetables at baseline. At the 2-year follow-up, the intervention group consumed 0.85 servings more than the delayed intervention group. The largest increases were observed among people 66 years or older (1 serving), those with education beyond high school (0.92 servings), those widowed or divorced (0.96 servings), and those attending church frequently (1.3 servings). The least improvement occurred among those aged 18 to 37 years and those who were single. The project was a successful model for achieving dietary change among rural African Americans.[171]

Therefore, in as much as it can be proven and documented that the local church has historically played a major role in the lives of those persons within the community, a foundation for community transformation through health awareness is warranted. The church must not allow the notion of individualism to invade its mission of outreach to the community as a whole. This is what Dr. James H. Harris meant when he challenged the church in his book *Pastoral Theology: A Black Church Perspective,*

> The black church is compelled to become an extroverted institution—one that will take more risks, demand more justice, and force blacks and whites to move beyond personal conversion to community

---

171 Marci Kramish Campbel, et al., "Fruit and Vegetable Consumption and Prevention of Cancer: the Black Churches United for Better Health Project," *American Journal of Public Health* 89, no. 9 (1999): 1390-1396.

transformation. To do this, it will have to change its focus of ministry.[172]

Dr. Harris' challenge to the black church may stand in direct opposition to the opinion of many in the United States of America as it relates to the issue of healthcare reform.

> The power of ethnocentrism—the belief that one's own ways are best—is illustrated by the recent debate over health care in the United States. In spite of repeated assertions that the United States system is 'the best in the world,' objective measures of infant mortality, life expectancy, and access to health care show that such assertions are false.[173]

"The current health care environment places emphasis on individual responsibility for health. Health behaviors may best be influenced in a community context."[174] Sherine Blagrove, a public health analyst, comments on the national issue of healthcare reform as it relates to the "safety net" within each community:

> The rising number of uninsured and the expansion of Medicaid managed care are straining the financial viability of the current health care safety net. The US health care system presents a troubling paradox: While perhaps the most sophisticated of any, it has among the worst health indices in the industrialized world. For millions, health care is available only through the largely public "safety net" of agencies

---

172 James H. Harris, *Pastoral Theology: A Black Church Perspective* (Minneapolis: Fortress Press, 1991), 35.

173 William Haviland, *Cultural Anthropology* (Fort Worth: Harcourt Brace College Publishers, 1996), 49.

174 Shirlee Drayton-Brooks, "Health promoting behaviors among African-American women with faith-based support," *The ABNF Journal* (September/October 2004).

organized specifically to serve the poor, uninsured, and otherwise vulnerable. Yet this network itself has become endangered, through shifting policies and lessened support. Funded by the US Department of Health and Human Services' Health Resources and Services Administration (HRSA), the IOM study attempted to capture the impact on safety net providers of waning political support, funding cuts, and the rapid expansion of managed care. It concluded that, in the absence of massive reforms, the safety-net delivery system could collapse. That such a collapse would compromise the health status of millions of Americans is clear. More than 34.5 million people in the United States fall below the official poverty line, for a staggering poverty rate of 12.7%. Our health care industry comprises approximately 14% of the gross domestic product, and health care expenditures exceed $1 trillion annually. Yet we are one of the few major industrialized nations that does not guarantee health insurance to all residents, leaving 44 million persons without coverage.[175]

John M. Perkins, founder of Voice of Calvary Health Center in rural Mississippi contends:

> Ultimately, the only solution to the health care crisis will be a national system of health care. It will be a challenge to design this system so that it does not turn into a huge, ineffective bureaucracy and so that it allows people to choose which doctors will treat them. Such a system should be developed so that local enterprises can supply the clinics and local people can be employed; after all, health care involves a lot of money and resources, and those resources should be put to work to develop the community. It is important that

---

175 Sherine Blagrove, "How Much Can the Safety Net Hold?" *Minority Health Today* (July 2000), 1.

there be a measure of community input and control
over its health care provider.[176]

Even though there is currently not a national healthcare system in
place within the United States, it is evident that the health promotion
must begin on the "grassroots" level within the rural communities
stemming from the local church. "According to Glanville and Porche,
by focusing planned community level health promotion strategies on
several aggregates, the intervention will manifest its outcome at the
community level."[177] The historical foundation of this project rests
upon the notion of empowerment through a focus group within the
community, because it is within the "community" that improved
health outcomes can be experienced. "Social support within the
context of faith communities appears to mediate specific mediators
of health."[178]

"Trusting relationships, open communication, safe, comfortable, and
familiar environments were identified as important considerations
when planning health promotion interventions for an African-
American faith community."[179]

A successful program that reaches out to African
Americans requires recruiting from local organizations within communities, such as churches, Head

---

176 John M. Perkins, *Beyond Charity: The Call to Christian Community
Development*, 114.
177 C. Glanville and D. Porche, "Community level health promotion to improve
the health status of African-Americans," *The Journal of Multicultural Nursing
and Health* (1998), 4, 6-10.
178 Van Olphen, A. Schultz, B. Israel, L. Chatters, L. Klem, E.Parker, and D.
Williams, "Religious involvement, social support, and health among African-
American women on the Eastside of Detroit," *Journal of General Internal
Medicine* (2003), 18, 549-557.
179 Shirlee Drayton-Brooks, "Health promoting behaviors among African-
American women with faith-based support," *The ABNF Journal* (September/
October 2004).

Start programs, day care and senior centers, and public health clinics. It also means sending recruiters to neighborhood gathering places such as diners, Laundromats, beauty parlors, and barbershops.[180]

"African Americans often seek help from churches where they feel cared for and safe from the debilitating effects of institutional racism. Unfortunately, choice can delay needed attention at medical centers regardless of whether research or standard care is opted for by patients."[181]

Research has led the writer to the following examples of Christian-based rural health centers: Voice of Calvary Family Health Center (VOCFHC) and The Myers Christian Family Health Center, both of Mississippi. As aforementioned, Voice of Calvary Family Health Center was founded by John Perkins in 1981 in response to the great need for health care in an impoverished community. This ministry, which is an independently operated federal health center, prides itself in offering affordable services to all within the community. Voice of Calvary Family Health Center[182] is a full service health ministry with services ranging from comprehensive primary health care for all ages, men, women, pediatrics, geriatrics, breast and cervical cancer services.

The Myers Foundation Christian Family Health Center, with several locations throughout rural Mississippi, was founded by the Rev. Dr. Ronald V. Myers, Sr., M.D. and his wife Sylvia Holmes-Myers in 1990. In an interview with the writer, Dr. Myers shared the reason

---

180 Ashing and K. Griva, "The recruitment of breast cancer survivors into cancer control studies; a focus on African-American women," *The Journal of the National Medical Association* (1999), 91, 255-260.

181 B.J. Gale and J.R. Erickson, "How race affects health services use by older women." *Health Care for Women, International* (1997): 18, 221-232.

182 www.vocm.org/health.html

for establishing this health ministry. "The Myers Foundation Christian Family Health Center was founded to demonstrate the Gospel of Jesus Christ through holistic ministry to the poor in rural America."[183] It is the mission of the Myers Foundation Christian Family Health Center to promote programs which "develop individuals, families and communities, empowering them to reach their full potential in Christ."[184] In addition to serving as the medical director for the facilities, Dr. Myers is also an ordained Baptist minister, a American Baptist medical missionary, and an accomplished jazz musician. His efforts to help educate poor people about the necessity of preventative medicine and maintaining healthy lifestyles have been highlighted in the national spotlight on programs such as ABC network's "Good Morning America" television show and "People" magazine to name a few.

Summary

Inasmuch as research has proven that the African-American church has historically responded to the needs of the community, it is the contention of the writer that this particular health awareness ministry model through information and inspiration is warranted now in the 21st century. The statistics within this chapter are indicative of the fact that the need is great, particularly among African-Americans for raising the level of health awareness within the community in order to help individuals make informed decisions that will lead to healthy outcomes. There is further evidence of rural parishes, churches, and other Christian ministries that are actively engaged in the development and implementation of successful full-service

---

183 An interview with Dr. Ronald V. Myers, Sr., M.D. conducted on January 29, 2006 by the writer.
184 www.myersfoundation.net

health care ministry models. However, it is the contention of the writer that the essence of what motivates people to go to the health centers, schedule an appointment with their family physician for a routine preventative check-up, or to make the daily decision to eat the right foods, get adequate rest and exercise, has been and will be the preaching of the Gospel.

Biblical Foundations

But Daniel purposed in his heart that he would not defile himself with the portion of the king's meat, nor with the wine which he drank: therefore he requested of the prince of the eunuchs that he might not defile himself. Now God had brought Daniel into favor and tender love with the prince of the eunuchs. And the prince of the eunuchs said unto Daniel, I fear my lord the king, who hath appointed your meat and your drink: for why should he see your faces worse liking than the children which are of your sort? Then shall ye make me endanger my head to the king. Then said Daniel to Melzar, whom the prince of the eunuchs had set over Daniel, Hananiah, Mishael, and Azariah, prove thy servants, I beseech thee, ten days; and let them give us pulse to eat, and water to drink. Then let our countenances be looked upon before thee, and the countenance of the children that eat of the portion of the king's meat: and as thou seest, deal with thy servants. So he consented to them in this matter, and proved them ten days. And at the end of ten days their countenances appeared fairer and fatter in flesh than all the children which did eat the portion of the king's meat. (Dan.1: 8-15)

Maintaining a lifestyle that includes eating the right foods can result in healthy outcomes that have a positive and holistic effect upon the total person, which includes the body, soul, and spirit. The Old Testament scriptural text taken from the book of Daniel offers a clear biblical foundation for the purpose of providing health awareness initiatives within the rural context of ministry. Since it is the aim of this project to focus upon the health outcomes of the total person/individual, one must consider the "life situation" and some pertinent exegetical components of this ancient biblical text and examine its relevance to the ministry model in question.

Life Situation of the Text

The Book of Daniel is described as "one of the most important prophetic books of the Old Testament, indispensable as an introduction to New Testament prophecy dealing with the "times of the Gentiles: the manifestation of the man of sin, the Great Tribulation, the second coming of Christ, the resurrection, and the judgments."[185] This biblical text depicts the life of Daniel the prophet, who "was taken to Babylon while yet a boy, together with three other Hebrew youths of rank—Hananiah, Mishael, and Azariah—at the first deportation of the people of Judah in the fourth year of Jehoiakim (604 B.C.). He and his companions were obliged to enter the service of the royal court of Babylon, on which occasion he received the Chaldean name Belteshazzar, according to the Eastern custom of taking a new name when a change takes place in one's condition of life, and more especially if his personal liberty is thereby affected."[186] It was during the period of the exile that the text in question was framed. This was a time when the Babylonian empire besieged Judah and its inhabitants and took them into captivity. Studies indicate that life for most Jews living in captivity during the Exile was somewhat comfortable. B.W. Anderson notes, "The lot of the exiles, among whom [Ezekiel] had

---

185 Merrill F. Unger, *The New Unger's Bible Dictionary*, (Chicago: Moody Press, 1988), 275.
186 Ibid, 274-275.

been living for several years before his call, was not as bad as might have been feared. Many of the Jews deported in 597 were skilled craftsmen whose labor was evidently in great demand in Babylonia."[187] J. Kenneth Kuntz asserts,

> Undoubtedly the Jews in Babylon suffered more mentally and spiritually than they did physically. Their physical situation was tolerable enough; they were permitted to live in agricultural communities of their own, build houses, assemble together, and even enter into commercial dealings. Some Jewish exiles who engaged in trade within this foreign land were quite successful.[188]

There seems to be strong connection between the Jewish exiles and rural agricultural communities. One of the main attractions of living in rural agricultural communities is the ability of individuals to plant their own gardens and grow their own fruits and vegetables, which can lead to healthy outcomes. This is what many of the Jews did during this exilic period. B. W. Anderson stated:

> Evidently it was easy enough for the exiles to accept Jeremiah's advice to build houses and plant gardens, to raise families, and to show interest in the welfare of the city in which they lived (Jer. 29: 4-7). So their life was fairly comfortable, even though many yearned to return to their homeland."[189]

---

187 Bernhard W. Anderson, *Understanding the Old Testament* 2nd edition, (Englewood Cliffs, NJ: Prentice-Hall, 1966), 362.

188 J. Kenneth Kuntz, *The People of Ancient Israel: An Introduction to Old Testament Literature, History, and Thought,* (New York: Harpers and Row Publishers, 1974), 357.

189 Bernhard W. Anderson, *Understanding the Old Testament* 2nd edition, 363.

Though the Jewish exiles lived fairly comfortably in Babylon, there was great concern and care for their spiritual heritage and foundations.

> The most serious adjustment that the Jews of Babylonia had to make was a religious adjustment. Their faith had been oriented to the land of Palestine, the inheritance Yahweh had given them, and to the Temple of Jerusalem, the place where Yahweh caused his "name" to dwell. The greatest danger was that in time the Jewish faith, torn from these historical moorings, would be drowned in the sea of Babylonian culture.[190]

However, this was not the case with Daniel and his three Hebrew friends. Daniel and his friends were able hold on to their spiritual heritage and keep themselves undefiled because of the fact that they had become self-disciplined. The text indicates that Daniel had "purposed in his heart" that he would not eat from the king's table. Daniel's refusal to eat the king's meat was not only a decision motivated by the fact that the king's food was defiled or "ethically or ritually" unclean, but because eating in the Hebrew heritage is a "calling". Rabbi Kerry M. Olitzky and Rabbi Daniel Judson in their book entitled *The Rituals and Practices of Jewish Life*, assert:

> Every time we eat a meal, we remind ourselves to whom we belong: our people, our land, our God. In the company of friends and family or by ourselves, we declare that nourishment is not just a gift, it is a calling. We may eat alone or in small groups, but we live in community, bound to our history and our

---

190 Ibid, 376.

future. Every act of eating is an act of communion and rededication to the mission of Israel.[191]

Daniel purposed in his heart to keep his diet, because these things had been instilled within him through the teachings of the Torah. Daniel and his three friends were taught in Genesis 1:29 that God originally intended for humans to eat a healthy diet consisting of fruits and vegetables, the very first provision of food. They were also taught that after the flood in Genesis 9:3, God permitted humanity to eat "every moving thing that lives…even as the green herb have I given you all things." "The integral connection between life and food is significant as it points to the fact that the God who has given life does everything possible to sustain this life."[192] What these young men were taught enabled and empowered them to stay with their diet and thus a healthy and holistic lifestyle. The underlying concept of this ministry model of health awareness is through preaching and teaching so that individuals can make the right choices and develop the discipline needed to remain faithful to it.

There is a strong connection between lives of Daniel and the notable African-American professor of botany and agriculture, George Washington Carver. Both of them were able to prosper because of the fact that they remained wholly committed to their Creator. John Perry in his book entitled, *Unshakable Faith*, states that "Carver infused everything he did with a sincere spiritual element. From his earliest days, Carver looked to his Creator to lead his life and work."[193] Both men had been taught the importance of prayer and

191 Rabbi Kerry M. Olitzky and Rabbi Daniel Judson, *The Rituals and Practices of Jewish Life*, (Woodstock, Vermont: Jewish Lights Publishing, 2002), 138.
192 L. Juliana M. Claassens, *The God Who Provides: Biblical Images of Divine Nourishment*, (Nashville: Abingdon Press, 2004), 25-26.
193 John Perry, *Unshakable Faith: Booker T. Washington and George Washington Carver*, (Sisters, Oregon: Multnomah Publishers, 1999), 362.

devotion. "Daniel…kneeled upon his knees three times a day, and prayed, and gave thanks before his God."[194] John Perry also notes:

> Carver was an early riser, often up by four in the morning to walk in the woods before sunrise. By nine o'clock he was in his laboratory in a building nearby. He often prayed briefly before entering the lab, "Open thou mine eyes that I may behold wondrous things out of thy law." My help cometh from the Lord who made heaven and earth and all that in them is.

Both men knew of the importance of eating a healthy diet consisting of natural foods. Carver is most noted for his work with the peanut and the sweet potato. In a hearing held on January 20, 1926 at the U.S. Capitol's House Ways and Means Committee:

> Carver testified that peanuts were part of a "natural diet" that was meant for everyone. "If you go to the first chapter of Genesis, we can interpret very clearly, I think, what God intended when he said, "Behold, I have given you every herb that bears seed upon the face of the earth, and every tree bearing a seed. To you it shall be meat." That is what he means about it. It shall be meat. There is everything there to strengthen and nourish and keep the body alive and healthy…If all other vegetables on earth were destroyed, a perfectly balanced ration with all of the nutrients in it could be made with the sweet potato and the peanut. From the sweet potato we get starches and carbohydrates, and from the peanut we get all the muscle-building properties."[195]

---

194 Dan. 6:10b
195 John Perry, *Unshakable Faith: Booker T. Washington and George Washington Carver*, 309-310.

Although it was a great challenge, these two men held fast to their personal convictions on health and spirituality and it proved to be most beneficial.

> The author of Daniel belonged to the Hasidim, whose religious faith demanded loyalty to the Torah at any cost. As we read the stories in chapters 1-6, we should keep in mind that he was speaking at a time when even the possession of a copy of the Torah was a capital offense. But even in foreign surroundings, where they were under great pressure to eat the king's sumptuous fare, they were faithful to the dietary regulations of the Jewish Torah.[196]

The Levitical codes of the Jewish Torah consisted of dietary laws and regulations found in Leviticus 11. According to Olitzky and Judson, this Jewish principle of self-discipline is identified as "kashrut":

> Kashrut is a spiritual dietary discipline that guides me in all that I eat, a system that makes me mindful of what I am doing. The word *kashrut* means, simply, "propriety" or "fitness." Kosher food means food that is "proper" or "fit" for consumption.[197]

While Daniel and his three Hebrew friends were in captivity, they were selected for service in the king's royal court. The preparation period for this level of service consisted of submission to traditions, customs, and foods of the king. "The king ordered some of the brightest and best young men to be brought to him to learn the language and be trained to serve in his palace. They were to be fed the sumptuous fare from the king's own table, with an abundance

---

196 Bernhard W. Anderson, Understanding the Old Testament 2nd edition, 540-541.
197 Rabbi Kerry M. Olitzky and Rabbi Daniel Judson, *The Rituals and Practices of a Jewish Life*, 41.

of fat-laden, unhealthy foods."[198] This could possibly include meats saturated in blood (Lev. 17:10), unclean meats (Lev. 11:13-20), or food that had sacrificed or dedicated to other deities. According to the text, it was Daniel's choice to obey his God by maintaining a healthy lifestyle free of defilement. For Daniel and his three friends, the issue of "defilement" was not only ethical and ritual, but practical. Daniel's concerned himself with what foods are most healthy and nourishing for the body in a practical way. This Jewish concept is called "shmiraf haguf." "What led me to no longer ingest foods harmful to my health was the journey of *shmirat haguf*, caring for the body."[199] Furthermore, Olitzky and Judson said "something had changed, however. My consciousness had been stimulated. I had become, for the first time, mindful of my diet…I had made the connection between eating and health. Taste was no longer a factor. I just wanted to take better care of my body."[200]

> Daniel along with Shadrach, Meshach, and Abednego, asked to be excused from partaking of the rich food and wine and allowed to consume a diet of vegetables and waters. The king's steward was reluctant to consent; afraid he would be punished if they were not as healthy as the other captives. Daniel persuaded him to test them for ten days and then see how their condition compared with the others.[201]

"The goal was peak performance, physically and mentally. The "control group," against whom Daniel and his friends could be compared, was

198 Reginald Cherry, M.D., *Healing Prayer: God's Divine Intervention in Medicine, Faith, and Prayer*, (Nashville, TN: Thomas Nelson Publishers, 1999), 51.

199 Rabbi Kerry M. Olitzky and Rabbi Daniel Judson, *The Rituals and Practices of a Jewish Life*, 51.

200 Ibid, 45.

201 Reginald Cherry, M.D., *Healing Prayer: God's Divine Intervention in Medicine, Faith, and Prayer*, 52.

the rest of the Hebrew trainees."[202] B. W. Anderson comments, "even though they ate nothing more than vegetables and water, they proved stronger than anyone else in the training program."[203]

> At the end of the ten-day test, Daniel and his friends looked better and were healthier than the young men who ate the king's food. So they were allowed to continue their vegetables-and-water diet. At the end of the training period, the healthy eaters were strong and fit as well as clearheaded and keen of mind. What a great example of the benefits of a carbohydrate-rich diet (the carbohydrates being vegetables and fiber).[204]

Physical Health

First, the selected biblical text clearly indicates that eating the right foods had a positive effect upon the health and well being of the physical body. Dr. George H. Malkmus, states, "food comprises only about four percent of the nutritional needs of the body! Yet without the right kinds of food prepared in the right manner the body is incapable of building strong, healthy, vital, vibrant cells and maintaining the body in superior health! Eating the wrong kinds of food or foods prepared in the wrong manner can create havoc in the body, clog up the body and cause all kinds of physical problems."[205] Daniel and his three friends where in better shape, physically than their Hebrew counterparts that ate the rich dainties of the king's palace. The text suggests that a person's physical appearance reflects what they eat.

---

202 Bob Deffinbaugh, Th.M, "Between a Rock and a Hard Place," www.bible.org, 7.
203 Bernhard W. Anderson, *Understanding the Old Testament*, 541.
204 Reginald Cherry, M.D., *Healing Prayer: God's Divine Intervention in Medicine, Faith, and Prayer*, 52.
205 Dr. George H. Malkmus, *Why Christians Get Sick?*, (Shippensburg, PA: Destiny Image Publishers, 1995), 93.

Daniel told the prince of the eunuchs "let our countenances be looked upon." "God's gifts of food reach the inner being—something that becomes visible in the face that shines with oil."[206] The text suggests that healthy eating and drinking biblically (i.e. fruits, vegetables, and water) assists one in attaining and maintaining positive physical wellness. Referencing Psalm 104:28-29, L. Juliana M. Claassens comments:

> God's gift of food extends beyond mere utilitarian value and expresses something of the generosity of God's gift. In verse 15, God's gift of food not only includes the daily bread to strengthen the human heart but also wine to gladden the heart and oil to make the face shine. God's gifts of abundance are there to bring joy to people, to make them strong, happy, and beautiful.[207]

It also suggests that abstinence from certain foods contributes to better health outcomes. "The idea that fasting improves a person's health and beauty is found also in the more or less contemporaneous Book of Judith (8:6-7) and in the slightly later Test. Twelve Patriarchs (Joseph 3:4)."[208]

> Fasting also brings about an energy boost. Most people eating the typical American diet have a toxic building within their cells. This results in the mitochondria (the energy factory inside each cell) being unable to effectively produce energy for the body. Over time, fatigue, irritability and lethargy set in. But when we fast, cellular waste is removed and cells can begin

---

206 L. Juliana M. Claassens, *The God Who Provides: Biblical Images of Divine Nourishment*, 26.

207 Ibid, 26.

208 Louis F. Hartman and Alexander A. DiLella, *The Anchor Bible: The Book of Daniel* vol. 23, (Garden City, NY: Doubleday and Co., Inc., 1978).

making energy again. Periodic, short-term fasting will also strengthen your immune system and help you live longer. As your body detoxifies, your skin will eventually become clearer, the whites of your eyes usually become whiter, and your mental functioning usually improves.[209]

Hilary Horton-Brown, staff nutritionist at Boise State University suggests for individuals to:

Maintain a diet high in antioxidants and energy when under stress. This means many fruits and vegetables that are rich and deep in color, plenty of lean dairy products and snacking throughout the day on mini-meals. Stay away from simple sugars such as pop and candy, because these things will trigger a cycle of high and low blood sugar and cause cravings for more sugar. Don't rely on caffeine to 'keep you going.' Get your energy from healthy foods. Don't forget to drink plenty of water. Dehydration leads to mental and physical fatigue.[210]

Daniel and his three friends chose to consume only water and fresh fruits and vegetables.

The body uses water to cleanse and remove toxins, to lubricate, to cool the body when overheated, etc. In fact, the body is comprised of from 75% to 85% water! For the proper functioning of the body to maintain health, to cleanse, or to heal, the body must have pure water![211]

---

209 Don Colbert, M.D., "Do you need Toxic Relief?" *Enjoying Everyday Life,* (Fenton, MO: Joyce Meyer Ministries, Inc., 2005), 22.

210 Hilary Horton-Brown with Anjie Robinson, *The Arbiter Online: Boise State's Independent Student Newspaper,* "Healthy Habits are key to getting a hold on midterm stress." (November 2003), www.arbiteronline.com.

211 Dr. George H. Malkmus, *Why Christians Get Sick,* 92.

"Finally, try to decrease such foods as caffeine, saturated fat, salt and sugar from your diet. Foods to increase to affect a healthy diet are fresh fruits, dietary fiber, vegetables and water."[212]

Mental and Emotional Health

Secondly, not only did consumption of healthy food and drink produce positive outcomes in the physical bodies of these four biblical young men, but the text suggests that eating right greatly enhanced the realm of the soul (i.e. mind, emotions, wisdom, decision-making abilities, etc.). The biblical text states that, "in all matters of wisdom and understanding, that the king enquired of them, he found them ten times better than all the magicians and astrologers that were in all his realm."[213]

> The term soul specifies that in the immaterial part of [humanity] that concerns life, action, and emotion. The Greek term *psuche* has the simple meaning of life; that in which there is life, a living being. It also has the meaning of the seat of the feelings, desires, affections, and aversions...[214]

These four young men were not stressed out, fatigued, and/or unable to perform. They were at "the top of their class." Eating the right foods caused the four Hebrew boys to prosper and excel in all that they went forth to accomplish. Studies have repeatedly proven that the human body functions best physically and mentally when receiving adequate nutrition and rest. "Since stress and poor nutrition often

---

212 Hilary Horton-Brown with Anjie Robsinson, *The Arbiter Online: Boise State's Independent Student Newspaper,* "Healthy Habits are key to getting a hold on midterm stress." (November 2003), www.arbiteronline.com.
213 Dan. 1:20
214 Merrill F. Unger, *The New Unger's Bible Dictionary*, 1213-1216.

go hand in hand, it is important to make sure to eat healthy…as well as making sure to eat at least three meals during the day to include breakfast. A person's body/mind needs energy after more than 8-12 hours without food. Skipping breakfast can make you tired and cause headaches."[215]

Spiritual Health and Well-being

The final component of the biblical foundation that addresses the ministry model in question is the effect upon the spirituality and prosperity of individuals within the rural context. Not only does health promotion produce positive results in the physical body and within the realm of the soul, (i.e. mind, emotions, wisdom, and decision-making), but healthy behaviors enhance the quality of one's spirituality. To further expound upon this notion, let's consider the New Testament biblical text taken from the second verse of the third epistle of John: "Beloved, I wish above all things that thou mayest prosper and be in health, even as thy soul prospereth." The third epistle of John "is addressed personally to Gaius, possibly the leader of a small church in Asia Minor."[216]

> He was probably a convert of St. John, and a layman of wealth and distinction in some city near Ephesus, A.D. after 90. The epistle was written for the purpose of commending to the kindness and hospitality of Gaius some Christians who were strangers in the place where he lived.[217]

---

215 Hilary Horton-Brown with Anjie Robsinson, *The Arbiter Online: Boise State Independent Student Newspaper*, "Healthy habits are key to getting a hold on midterm stress", www.arbiteronline.com

216 J. B. Phillips, *Letters to Young Churches: A translation of the New Testament Epistles*, (New York: The MacMillan Co., 1961), 221.

217 Merrill F. Unger, *The Unger's Bible Dictionary*, 451.

"These "brothers and sisters" or "the holy and beloved" gathered in the homes of more prosperous members, such as those of Gaius in Corinth, Nympha in Laodicea, or Philemon at Colossae."[218]

> In one community a certain Diotrephes, who has emerged as a leader, has decided to keep out traveling missionaries including those from the presbyter. His refusal of hospitality causes the presbyter to write III John to Gaius, seemingly a wealthy person in a neighboring community. Gaius has been providing hospitality on a temporary basis, but the presbyter wants him to take over larger responsibilities for helping the missionaries, including the well-known Demetrius, who will soon arrive.[219]

"John prays that the letter may find Gaius as prosperous and healthy in body as he apparently is in soul. John was very happy when Christians brought news that Gaius was a truly consecrated man and living a Christian life."[220] "A health wish is also a feature in the opening of secular letters, but the presbyter extends his concerns to Gaius' spiritual welfare—a connection of soul and body."[221] This notion of promoting healthy lifestyles should also include the health and prosperity of the "total" or "whole" being: body, soul, and spirit. It is evident that this New Testament biblical text promotes physical, mental, and spiritual health and well being.

> Although a great many people assume that the Bible is strictly a religious book dealing exclusively with

---

218 Gayla Visalli, ed., *After Jesus, The Triumph of Christianity*, (Pleasantville, NY: Reader's Digest Association, Inc., 1992), 101.

219 Raymond E. Brown, *An Introduction to the New Testament*, (New York: Doubleday & Co., 1997), 401.

220 Francis Bayard Rhein, *An Analytical Approach to the New Testament*, (Woodbury, NY: Barron's Educational Services, Inc., 1966), 356.

221 Raymond E. Brown, *An Introduction to the New Testament*, 401.

"spiritual" matters, even a casual study of the scriptures reveals that they deal with [humanity] as a whole person—body, mind, and spirit. The biblical text is largely directed to nurturing, protecting, and guiding human begins to achieve their full potential in every area of their being. For example, biblical scholars have determined that one out of three Old Testament laws dealt with issues of health. Although the purpose of those laws may not have been fully understood at the time they were established, we now know that each was carefully designed to make a definite, positive contribution to [humanity's] well-being."[222]

The underlying foundational theme in the III John 1:2 text is this: health promotion is for the whole being. The opening salutation of John to Gaius speaks of "prosperity" and "health", which is not uncommon in secular letters as well.

The Greek term for "prosper" is "euodoo" which means to help on one's way (eu, "well", hodos, "a way or journey"), is used in the passive voice signifying "to have a prosperous journey,"…in material things; the continuous tense suggests the successive circumstances of varying prosperity as week follows week; in III John 1:2, of the "prosperity" of physical and spiritual health.[223]

"The Greek term for health "hugianio" denotes to be healthy, sound, in good health, i.e. sound, whole."[224] This is a clear indication of the relationship between health and prosperity as it relates to the

---

222 Reginald Cherry, M.D., *Healing Prayer: God's Divine Intervention in Medicine, Faith, and Prayer*, 46-47.

223 W.E. Vine, *Vine's Complete Expository Dictionary of Old and New Testament Words*, (Nashville: Thomas Nelson Publishers, 1985), 495.

224 Ibid, 295.

well-being of the total person. Rev. Dr. Tom Droege, director of the Interfaith Health Program at the Carter Center comments that:

> Linking health care to spirituality is not a modern discovery. So wedded is health to spiritual life that the first professional health care advisors were doctor/priests who interceded with the deities or interpreted divine will as expressed in dreams and visions.[225]

Summary

In conclusion, it has been the attempt of the writer to lift up two biblical texts taken from Old and New Testaments showing the relationship of the ministry model: Equipping and Empowering Rural Church leaders in 21st Century Ministry through Health Awareness. The Old Testament text taken from Daniel provides a biblical basis for doing an action research project on a small cell group within the ministry context for the promotion of healthy outcomes in the lives of the participants. Research has led the writer to believe that the Exile spoken of in the Old Testament may have given birth to small support/cell groups that could have led to the beginning of the synagogue. According to B. W. Anderson:

> In the Exile, then, the people realized that they could turn to God anywhere with confidence that he would be near, and that he would be their sanctuary in a foreign land. Moreover, during this period Jews undoubtedly came together in small groups, after the manner of the elders who consulted Ezekiel in his house, to be instructed in their scriptural traditions and to worship informally. It has often been suggested that the synagogue, "gathering together" (as the Greek

---

225 Rev. Richard B. Gilbert, ed., *Healthcare and Spirituality: Listening, Assessing, Caring* (Amityville, NY: Baywood Publishing Co., 2002), iii.

word "synagogue" means) for worship and teaching,
may have originated during the Exile.[226]

Furthermore, the "health" wish and admonishment to provide
servant-leadership/hospitality to other Christians issued by John to
the wealthy and prosperous church leader Gaius, provides a biblical
basis for empowering rural church leaders in the ministry context to
realize the importance of serving within the community. In addition,
it provides a challenge to the church and rural church leaders to
examine their own health conditions, because effective ministry is
accomplished when the individuals doing ministry are functioning
at their best level of health and prosperity.

---

226 Bernhard W. Anderson, *Understanding the Old Testament* 2nd ed., 378.

CHAPTER FOUR

Methodology

THIS CHAPTER WILL ADDRESS THE methodology that was used in the development of a health awareness ministry model through preaching and teaching. The ministry model that is developed in this section will be implemented at the Jerusalem Baptist Church of Temperanceville, Virginia, which is located on Virginia's Eastern Shore. The results of the model's implementation will be expounded upon in the following chapter of this work. The research methodology and the design of the model of ministry to be used in the field experience will be discussed in this chapter.

The period of designing the ministry model began in the fall of 2004. A general church survey[227] was distributed among several members of the Jerusalem Baptist Church. The purpose of the survey was for the writer to attain a better understanding of the type of problem statement that would need to be addressed. The results of the general church survey or "needs assessment" indicated that the preaching and teaching ministry was a major strength of the church. Many of the church members were very satisfied with their church

---

227 A copy of this survey is located in Appendix G.

home, but felt that they could become better equipped for ministry holistically.

Following a collaborative dialogue with context associates, mentors, and peer associates, the following problem statement was formulated by the writer. The overall problem to be addressed within this context of ministry is the fact that this particular rural church is currently unprepared and ill-equipped for ministry to the church and community in the 21st Century regarding health awareness and health education.

Hypothesis

The hypothesis of this ministry model is that rural church leadership within this particular context will become better equipped and prepared for 21st Century ministry and leadership through health awareness with the implementation of the following objectives. The objectives of the ministry project are two-fold. The first objective is to increase the level of awareness of the importance of the need for 21st Century ministry as it relates to health education and awareness within the rural church and community. The second objective is to provide a selective focus group of church leaders the practical tools needed to change lifestyle habits that will result in a positive influence upon their health. Thus, these church leaders would not only become better informed, but better equipped, physically, mentally, and spiritually to carry out ministry and leadership responsibilities within the church.

Intervention

There are three primary components of the actual ministry project. The first component of the intervention or treatment was increasing the level of health awareness of the rural congregation and church leadership through the preachment. Three relevant and practical sermons[228] were preached during the 8:00 A.M. and 11:00 A.M. worship experiences. The second component of the treatment included the institution of a church-wide health awareness season through the establishment of a focus group of participants. The participants would be exposed to practical tools needed to change lifestyle habits relating to health such as a Bible Study packet/booklet compiled by the writer entitled, "Health and Wellness: Equipping and Empowering The Church through Health Awareness in Body, Soul, and Spirit." A major portion of the bible study packet included information pertaining to the implementation of the "Body and Soul Program: A Celebration of Healthy Eating and Living" aforementioned in the second and third chapters of this work. The focus group was also exposed to a "Healthy Eating and Nutrition Seminar" held at the church and conducted by the Accomack County Cooperative Extension Office of Accomac, Virginia. The third component of the treatment was the development and implementation of a "Forty-Day Prayer and Consecration Fast" which began on Ash Wednesday March 1, 2006 and lasted throughout the duration of the Lenten season. The purpose of the corporate fast, in addition to the observance of the passion of Christ, was to promote healthy eating habits, consumption of more fruits and vegetables, natural colon cleansing, and a well-balanced healthy lifestyle of prayer, meditation, and consecration. The events of the health awareness season were recorded in the March 4, 2006 edition of the *Eastern Shore News*.

---

228 Manuscripts of the three sermons preached during health awareness season are located in Appendices H, I, J.

Research Design

The research methodology used in this ministry project was quantitative as opposed to qualitative. The overall design of the study utilized the experimental method of research. "An experimental method discussion follows a standard form: participants, materials, procedures, and measures."[229] More specifically, the type of experimental procedure used was the "pre-experimental one group pre-test-post-test design." (See Table 1)

Table 1

$$O_1\text{--------------} X \text{--------------} O_2$$

"With pre-experimental designs, the researcher studies a single group and provides an intervention during the experiment. This design does not have a control group to compare with the experimental group."[230]

The participants, a focus group consisting of rural African-American church leaders, were initially measured on a pre-test instrument. A pre-program survey accompanied the pre-test instrument. The participants were then exposed to the aforementioned treatment then measured again on a post-test instrument, which consisted of the National Health Test. The post-test instrument was also accompanied by a post-program survey administered by the writer.

---

229 John W. Creswell, *Research Design: Qualitative, Quantitative, and Mixed Methods Approaches* 2nd edition, (Thousand Oaks, CA: Sage Publications, Inc., 2003), 162.
230 Ibid, 167.

Measurement and Instrumentation

The participants measured were obtained through a non-random selection process. The forty participants consisted of a naturally found bible study group of church leaders with age ranges from (14-86). The instrumentation utilized was the "National Health Test: the first step for Americans on the path to weight-loss and wellness." The instrument consists of ten simple questions, graded on a 10-point scale to determine the overall level of an individual's personal health awareness. The writer selected this particular instrument because of its simplicity and the fact that it would not be difficult to administer to the participants. The test can be taken online through the internet, or manually through a DVD presentation that explains the questions. Verbal permission was granted by the staff of Dr. Julian Whitaker, M.D., developer of the instrument and owner and operator of the Whitaker Wellness Institute, Inc.

Dr. Julian Whitaker, M.D. is a 1966 graduate of Dartmouth College and received his medical training at Emory University Medical School in Atlanta, Georgia in 1970. Dr. Whitaker is a member of the American Medical Association and is board certified in anti-aging medicine. He is the author of 10 books including *Reversing Heart Disease* and *Reversing Diabetes*. He operates the largest, most comprehensive alternative medicine clinic in the United States of America, having served more than 35,000 patients. Dr. Julian Whitaker, M.D. developed the National Health Test instrument in collaboration with *USA Today Weekend*, Highland Video & Entertainment, and Associated Television, Inc. with a DVD presentation hosted by Bryant Gumble. Authorization and limited license to administer the test and exhibit the DVD was granted by Associated Television, Inc.

CHAPTER FIVE

Field Experience

THIS CHAPTER WILL DISCUSS WHAT actually occurred during the implementation of the ministry project. The writer will further expound upon the objectives of the project. There will also be a section devoted to data collection, data analysis, and the overall results of the ministry model.

As stated earlier within this document, the objectives of the ministry project included: increasing the level of awareness of the importance of the need for 21st century ministry as it relates to health awareness within the rural community through the treatment of preaching three relevant sermons and providing a selective focus group the practical tools needed to change habits that would result in a positive influence upon their health.

Prior to the implementation of the project goals and objectives, the writer had to address a few minor obstacles. Some of the church members expressed a reluctance to participate in a "health test" at the church due to fear. Some were apprehensive about the health awareness project, because they thought that they would have to physically undress at the church or that they would be personally exposed to the pastor/writer. Some went home to discuss the possibility of participating with their adult children, many of whom felt that this was unnecessary. After the misunderstandings were cleared up and the objectives of the project were explained in detail and put in writing, many of the members were more inclined to participate in the ministry project.

Prior to implementation of the treatment, the pre-test instrument was administered to forty participants between the ages of 14 and 86 on February 22, 2006. The pre-test instrument was administered anonymously to encourage honesty in answering the health questions. The participants were assigned an identification number synonymous with their date of birth. The average score of the forty participants was 67%. According to the grading scale of the National Health Test developed by Dr. Julian Whitaker, M.D., 67% is the equivalent of a "D" for denial of living a healthy lifestyle. This information proved that there was a great need for more awareness.

The forty participants underwent a treatment period of forty days, where they were exposed to three relevant sermons on health awareness preached by the researcher: "He's A Keeper", "Under New Management", and "Dealing with Depression." Each of the three sermons was preached during the 8 A.M. and 11 A.M. Sunday morning worship experiences. A few of the participants commented on the affect of the preaching series. Some of the comments included: "It encouraged me to be more concerned about my health", "All very helpful…reminds me that my body is a temple and I should take care of it to live to the fullest", "It helped me in a way, because I did not know how to deal with depression at that time, but I know now", and "It has allowed me to see that you have to be careful of the food that you eat, and how important your health can be."

A practical bible study on health awareness as it relates to the three-fold nature of humanity: body, soul, and spirit was taught by the writer. A portion of the materials found within the bible study packet included information from the "Body and Soul: A Celebration of Healthy Eating", a program originating from similar research conducted by the Black Churches United for Better Health of North Carolina. The focus group was also exposed to a community-wide "Healthy eating and Nutrition Seminar" conducted at the church by the Accomack County Cooperative Extension Office on March 16, 2006. The seminar was conducted from 7:00 P.M. to 9:00 P.M. by Ms. Susan O'Brien, coordinator of the nutrition program. There were nineteen attendees and each person received handouts, health brochures, and free hot soup, fresh salad and juice. Participants had an opportunity to receive door prizes and incentives for attending the seminar. Conducting an on site seminar was done to bring the information to the participants in an atmosphere where they could receive the information as well as be comfortable. One participant commented, "The seminar could have included more menus for healthy cooking."

A forty-day prayer and consecration "Daniel Fast" was conducted throughout the health awareness season to promote healthy eating and increased consumption of fruits and vegetables. The "Daniel Fast' was also opened up to the community and general public and was well received by many. A large percentage of the church members participated in the fast, as well as several individuals from other states and regions to include North Carolina, South Carolina, Georgia, Pennsylvania, and the US Virgin Islands. One participant commented saying, "I went down two dress sizes as a result of the 40-day fast."

Some of the original forty participants "dropped-out" of the ministry project either mid-way or toward its completion due to scheduling conflicts, employment changes, lack of interest, and unknown reasons. The post-test instrument was given on May 3, 2006 and May 10, 2006 to a total of twenty-four remaining participants. The reason that the post-test was administered on two different dates was due to the fact that many of the participants were absent on May 3, 2006, therefore after a general announcement was made from the pulpit by the writer, the remainder of the participants were tested on May 10, 2006. Sixteen of the twenty-four participants were female. Six of the twenty-four participants were male. Two of the twenty-four participants did not answer the gender question.

It was estimated by the writer that the greatest participation would be from the female population. Based on the "North Carolina" research project as well as "Body and Soul" it is proven. Male participation in health activities, in addition to church activities are limited in number. It is possible that regardless of the identification system, there were two individuals that did not want to be identified by the researcher for various reasons, which may include but not be limited to gender bias.

Results Comparison by Gender

Results of the ministry model indicate that the males showed signs of improvement after taking the post-test, however the females somewhat remained the same overall. The two participants that did not answer the gender question exhibited great improvement by 8%. The female population attempted to make greater efforts than the male population during the entire project. The female population displayed the effort to gather, memorize and practice more of the tools and information that was shared by the researcher. The results of the pre-test indicate that the male population is limited. The unknown gender participants scored lower than both populations.

Educational levels of the participants

Twelve of the twenty-four participants were high school graduates or GED recipients. Four of the twenty-four participants had some college background. Four of the twenty-four participants had some high school education. Two of the twenty-four participants were currently enrolled in high school. Two of the twenty-four participants did not answer the education question.

Health and education in relation to work and work benefits could be a determining factor in the results of the ministry model. Those that work a trade, retail, or are self- employed usually are affected differently than those that do not. Examining the data closely shows that the majority of the participants were High School Graduates. The knowledge of various types of available health programs gives one the ability to make the most informed decisions.

Results comparison by Educational Level

Pre and Post test results repeatedly reveal that the current high school students had the highest scores on the National Health Test. The post-test scores of those with "less than a high school education" actually decreased by 6%. The two participants that did not answer the education question on the pre-test, actually exhibited an increased awareness by 8%.

Student scores will, for the most part be highest due to the fact that physical activity is required of them through sports and physical education classes. Student's meals are planned by qualified school nutritionists, sports physicals are also required by the athletic director in order to participate in both varsity and junior varsity athletics. Participants with less than a High School education experienced a decrease in scores because the opportunity to retrieve information from officials on the Secondary Education level was limited. The two unknown participants that did not answer the question may have considered themselves "outliers" in the project, which is a term for people that exceed or subset the outlined qualifications for participants within the program.

Results Comparison by Generation

The scores of the participants were divided in generations according to age ranges. Those participants between the ages of 14-19 are classified as "youth." Those participants between the ages of 20-35 are classified as "young adults." Those participants between the ages of 36-54 are classified as "middle-aged." Those participants that are age 55 and above are classified as "senior-citizens." The senior citizen participants averaged a higher score than the other generations during the pre-test, but their scores decreased to 66% after the post-test. The young adult participants averaged a higher score than the other generations after the post-test and exhibited the highest rate of improvement and increased health awareness.

Youth are monitored therefore; their scores were higher at the onset of the project and slowly dwindled. Young adults are pre-occupied with "day to day living", everyday needs, the essentials of food, clothing, and shelter. After taking the Pre-test the young adult participants saw the importance of health awareness and were able to show the highest rate of improvement and increase their health awareness. Between the ages of 36 and 54 years old health is more of a concern. Due to age, senior citizens are limited in the amount of work they can do. Enjoyment of the quality of life is essential in the "golden years". Health is pinnacle to senior citizens. Finding the best physicians, therapists, and nurses and pharmacists are important for this group. Pharmacists that are well versed and able to explain the dosage and side effects of prescribed medications are also a part of the concern of senior citizens.

54% of the remaining participant's scores actually increased. 42% of the remaining participant's scores decreased. One individual's score remained the same. The average score of the participants taking the post-test was 70%, which is the equivalent of a "C" for a need to be concerned for one's health. The fact that the overall average increased one by grade level is an indication that the objectives of the overall ministry project were achieved and that there was a marginal attitudinal change among the participants as it relates to the level of health awareness within the ministry context.

It is the contention of the writer that several factors could attribute to the reason why the data reflects marginal attitudinal change. First of all, it could be that many of the participants did not agree with the curriculum used and thereby rejected the information that was taught. Secondly, some of the participants did not share the same practices and beliefs as the person that designed the instrument. For instance, many of the participants responded to the question on alcoholic beverages, stating that they do not consume them. However, according to the instrumentation, the consumption of certain alcoholic beverages is vital and necessary for maintaining a healthy heart. Third, it can be suggested that due to the high rate of illiteracy on Virginia's Eastern Shore, that some perhaps did not fully understand the questions, even though they were given both orally and in literary form. Finally, it is the suspicion of the writer, that even though the instrument was administered anonymously there are a few that still did not answer the questions honestly because they may have thought that the writer could identify them according to their date of birth. This suspicion is especially warranted due to the fact that the project was conducted in a small rural church context, where everyone is connected.

Summary

The objective of chapter five was to state what occurred when the health awareness ministry model was implemented at the Jerusalem Baptist Church of Temperanceville. The model design was an extremely intensive and time-consuming event. The overall process sought to raise the level of health awareness within the congregation in order to affect change within the community as a whole. The model design, though directed toward the rural church leaders and members of the focus group, was also implemented for the benefit of the entire rural community on Virginia's Eastern Shore. The ministry model was implemented during one of the busiest times on the Christian calendar, the Lenten season. A portion of the ministry model was briefly interrupted due to Lenten and Holy Week services. However, the results indicate that the objectives were met, there was marginal attitudinal change, though there was an increase in the overall average scores of the participants that remained in the ministry project.

CHAPTER SIX

Reflection, Summary, and Conclusion

PRIOR TO THE IMPLEMENTATION OF the ministry model, the pastor, officers, and members of the Jerusalem Baptist Church were unequipped and unprepared for effective and meaningful ministry in the 21st century, as it relates to health awareness. Poor nutrition, unhealthy eating habits, lack of physical activity, and an abundance of stress plagued the members of the ministry context in question. The need for an increase in awareness and lifestyle transformation was of utmost importance within this ministry project, if the direction of this particular rural church would change for the better. This is supported by the results of the pre-test, which indicate an average score of 67% attainted by the participants on the National Health Test. This score fell in the "D" range which is next to the lowest ranking score on the scale. The hypothesis of the writer was proven and the steps toward implementation began.

Before the intervention was implemented to affect change upon the selected participants, there were some minor problems that needed to be addressed. First, it was very difficult for the writer to solicit participation in the ministry project. It is the writer's suspicion, that many people were either afraid to find out about their health status or they already knew about their negative health status but did not want anyone else to know. Some were reluctant to participate because they felt that the writer/pastor would be privy to personal information about their physical health and lifestyle habits. For instance, many did not want the pastor/writer to know that they were smokers and/or occasionally drank alcoholic beverages. In order to address this, the potential participants were told that they could participate without giving their names. Their scores could be reported by a "code" containing their birthdates. This would encourage the participants to answer the questions honestly. As stated in the previous chapter, some felt that they would have to physically undress at the church and that the pastor/writer would conduct the physical. After assuring the potential volunteers that a physical could only be provided by a licensed physician and that no one would have to physically undress, many were more willing to participate in the ministry project, especially the senior citizens.

The ministry project was implemented on Ash Wednesday March 1, 2006, but many of the participants did not complete the program for various reasons. Some were just not interested in the content matter and others had scheduling and job conflicts at night when the events actually occurred. Looking back in retrospect, the writer would have liked to have had two different groups of participants, exposed to the same treatment, one during the day and the other group during the evening, however time would not permit. It is also the opinion of the writer that if the project were conducted at a time of the year, other than the busy Lenten season, many perhaps would have remained in the program. However, due to scheduling conflicts, Holy Week and Lenten services, the project was forced to alternate weeks and certain events were postponed.

If this ministry project were replicated and conducted elsewhere, it would be the suggestion of the writer that transportation be provided to the sessions. Oftentimes in the rural context of ministry, public transportation is rarely available. Some participants were relying upon other individuals for a ride to the church and back home. Others were unable to attend the session with consistency due to poor transportation, automobile troubles, and the price of fuel at the time of the project implementation. Another consideration for future replication of this ministry model would be the issue of timing. Due to the rapid pace of the Doctor of Ministry program, it is the opinion of the writer that more time would be needed to adequately address the needs of the participants, interact with other guest speakers and experts from the health community, and explore the many dimensions of health awareness.

As noted in the previous chapter, the treatment included the preaching of three relevant sermons on health awareness, a practical bible study on health and wellness which included the implementation of the "Body and Soul" program, a healthy eating and nutrition seminar, and a forty-day consecration fast to encourage the consumption of at least five to nine fruits and vegetables per day. A few of the comments from the participants during the post-test indicated that the preaching was effective. However, the writer would suggest the development of an illustrated sermon, where individuals can physically focus on different fruits, vegetables, and other health information spoken of in the Bible. Also, a sermon which specifically addresses the "diet" as spoken of in the book of Daniel would have been a great tool for strengthening the overall results of the project. A large portion of the Bible Study packet included information from the "Body and Soul" program. This is clearly a program that would be of greater value and benefit to the rural church on an extended basis.

More time would be needed to see the fulfillment of that particular program.

The forty-day fast was a tremendous success because not only did it encourage healthy eating habits and the consumption of the recommended five to nine fruits and vegetables per day, but it also provided spiritual strength, wisdom, and guidance to the congregation as a whole. Many of the concepts for the forty-day fast were gleaned from *T.G.I.F. Thank God I'm Fasting*, an insightful and practical book by Dr. Joan L. Wharton who also served as a professional associate to the writer in the development of this ministry model. The writer also recommends *God's Chosen Fast: A Spiritual and Practical Guide to Fasting* by Arthur Wallis as an excellent foundational teaching aid on healthy fasting practices in a 21st century world.

The ministry project was a success and increased health awareness was achieved. This was supported by the results of the post-test in which the average score went from 67% "D" to 70% "C". However, the results could have been better if the following conditions were met. First of all, adequate and appropriate space for physical fitness activities to be conducted. The church did not have a gymnasium or multi-purpose rooms with flooring to withstand physical fitness classes or intense exercising. The weather conditions were not conducive for outdoor physical training during that particular season of the year. Secondly, there could have been some funding allocated in the church ministries budget for the implementation of the program. This would have offset the cost of field trips, gifts, incentives and other outings held to encourage healthy lifestyles. Perhaps in the development of future health awareness ministries within the local church, a partnership or collaboration should be formed between the local Y.M.C.A., Curves, Parks and Recreation, or other institutions promoting healthy lifestyles through physical fitness. Thirdly, the writer would have liked to have had more one-on-one time with the participants to find out their individual needs so that the program could address specific sicknesses, ailments, and infirmities as well as preventative measures.

Future Implications Within the Ministry Context

This ministry project has led to further exploration into the "Body and Soul" program as well as the development of a health ministry at the church. A partnership has been established with the local chapter of the American Cancer Society South Atlantic Division, Inc. which serves Delaware, Georgia, Maryland, North Carolina, South Carolina, Virginia, West Virginia, and Washington, D.C. Within this collaborative effort, recruited individuals within the ministry context will be trained to serve as facilitators for the Body and Soul program/health ministry of the local congregation. It is also worth noting that the congregation has started to offer more of a healthier selection of food and drink during the significant annual services such as Homecoming Sunday and Church Anniversary. The culinary committee has also included turkey bacon, sausages, and fresh fruit trays in addition to serving traditional pork dishes during prayer breakfast services. They have also started serving fresh salads with the traditional refreshments during afternoon services. This is a great indication that health awareness has been increased in the hearts and minds of those that prepare the food for church functions.

Finally, not only has the ministry context been impacted by this health awareness project, but the writer has been further equipped and empowered in 21st century ministry through holistic health and wellness. As ministers lead their faith communities, they lead by example and setting a good example in their health habits will have a positive impact upon the lives of the parishioners and their lives as well. The writer's health habits have changed significantly. In addition to healthy eating and considering the nutritional value of fruits and vegetables, the writer has also begun to examine the larger picture of life and ministry, developing the ability to balance church, ministry, family, career, and live life to the fullest. One of the greatest rewards of this Doctor of Ministry project is seeing those rural church leaders, officials, members, and participants impacted by the lifestyle changes of the writer/pastor that it causes them to consider implementing change as well. The writer/pastor shared with the congregation that in addition to healthy choices in body, soul, and spirit, he has begun to take care of himself by going to the local "wellness spa." The writer's excitement invoked a great response from the people within the context, and now many of the church members are inquiring about how to set an appointment at the day spa so that they can be happy, healthy and feel well.

Recommendations for Future Research

It is the recommendation of the writer that perhaps this work may lead to some future research pertaining to health awareness among clergy and specifically those in pastoral leadership. It is evident that those key leaders and individuals in ministry can not and will not be effective in ministry if they are not healthy and well taken care of. In the process of writing this final document, the wife of the writer experienced a traumatic illness which was triggered by lack of stress-management and could have been avoided. That is when this ministry project really became even more personal to the writer. When this illness occurred, it caused the writer to understand more fully the notion of "action research." It's one thing to stand back and observe the actions and reactions of the subjects being researched, but it is something to grapple with when the issue has come to one's front door. Perhaps there should be some further exploration into the eating and physical fitness habits of African-American pastors, clergypersons and their spouses that serve in ministry by their side. If anything this ministry project, has encouraged the writer to take full advantage of every opportunity to live a healthy lifestyle, enjoy and live life to the fullest, and take advantage of every opportunity to walk in wellness and holistic ministry. Clergy persons should have hobbies, favorite pastimes that involve physical activity, and other enjoyable moments that promote health and wellness while engaging in ministry. This includes getting proper rest, nutritious meals, and a certain amount of physical fitness. It also means developing a good understanding of what counts most in life and making time for one's self in prayer and meditation. It goes without saying, if church leaders are not walking in holistic health, how will be they be able to maintain a level of quality and effective ministry to others whom they are serving.

This project also "opened the door" to the perils of depression that could possibly plague even those in the pulpit or engaging in pastoral caregiving or church leadership ministries. Perhaps further study could be done in this area, specifically relating to clergypersons throughout the world.

Conclusion

Due to the drastic increase in health disparities coupled with government cutbacks caused by an unstable and uncertain economy, it is the contention of the writer that the rural community that will suffer greatly. It is the suggestion of the writer that the appropriate response to the need which will continue to become so great would include several key points to be discussed now.

First, there is a need for more effective collaboration among rural churches and rural church leadership. More can be accomplished when the resources of several churches located within a certain radius of these rural communities are combined together. A collaborative effort among rural churches would promote healthy fellowship and networking within the community. The establishment of alliances will enable and empower small rural ministries to accomplish the "greater works than these" that Christ spoke of in the New Testament. One of the major concerns of some rural ministries is the fact that financial resources are limited. Rural churches must pool their resources together in this 21st century in order to address health awareness issues more effectively. Grant funding is available in many rural areas that have been identified as "underserved" communities. Foundations, institutions, and perhaps, the federal government would be more apt to awarding grant funding to those rural ministries that have the ability, resources, and number of people required to effectively administer a health program. Historically, many rural churches have collaborated for special services, certain community efforts, and the holiday events. An alliance of rural churches could possibly lead to the establishment of a health and wellness center, an urgent care/emergency center, or the employment of a full-time rural parish nurse to address the needs of those in the underserved areas.

Second, the rural church must strive to develop partnerships with the various institutions that help promote health and wellness within the community. Local hospitals, county health departments, grocery stores, and cooperative extension agencies to name a few are excellent resources for establishing partnerships to assist in achieving greater health awareness within rural communities. There is a wealth of information available to the public pertaining to nutrition, prevention, and physical fitness as well as individuals who are being compensated to educate and inform the public as well as unite with public institutions such as local schools and churches. These partnerships should not only be limited to the local hospitals and health departments, but churches should also seek to involve those within the private sector or those within the "marketplace" such as Gold's Gym, Curves, and the YMCA. In some cases, rural churches lack adequate facilities for exercise and physical fitness. Establishing partnerships within the "marketplace" would not only provide the right kind of facilities and equipment, but also healthier outcomes at a discounted rate.

Third, with the onset of government cut-backs to the rural community on the rise, rural churches can make a difference within their community through agricultural empowerment. Many of these underserved rural areas have the land, tools, and the knowledge of how to produce healthy crops of fruits and vegetables. Utilizing all of the God-given gifts and resources that are available and at disposal of the community, churches should be able to work together planting their own gardens, which would promote the healthy consumption of fruits and vegetables at a discounted rate, if not free. Historically, this is how many African-Americans have survived throughout the Reconstruction period and beyond. Perhaps, it may be time to go back to the basics.

Finally, it has been the aim of this final document to promote the importance of health awareness through the vehicle of inspiration and information. It is the writer's argument that religious commitment, spirituality, and health overall, have been and always will be intertwined. In order to for significant improvements in relation to health disparities in the rural community to take place, an awesome responsibility rests upon the preacher and the leaders of the rural church. The preacher is not only challenged to deliver a word that is relevant and effective for health awareness, but there is a great need for creativity within the ministries of the church. As proven within this final project, there may a significant percentage of individuals that reject or dismiss the information about health that is brought to them for various reasons. Today's rural pastor must attempt to reach the people where they are and continuously model the desired behavioral and attitudinal changes desired.

In addition to leading by example, the rural pastor can spread this message of health awareness and spirituality to those that are currently un-churched. From this perspective, the writer asserts that this health awareness model can become an effective evangelistic strategy to reach the un-churched with an issue that is relevant to their everyday lifestyle. This may involve the development of a quarterly health newsletter, a health empowerment minute with the pastor on the local radio station, a monthly excerpt on health and spirituality in the local newspaper, or perhaps an emailed devotional of the day which incorporates health and spirituality. In addition to promoting health awareness, the church would be fulfilling the Great Commission of Christ which states, "Go ye therefore and teach all nations…" This message of hope, health, and healing for the nations has become an area of importance that the will propel the church into its proper place of influence—at the forefront of this society affecting change and transformation in this 21st Century.

JERUSALEM BAPTIST CHURCH
10011 JERUSALEM ROAD P.O. BOX 26
TEMPERANCEVILLE, VA 23442
REV. MICHAEL THOMAS SCOTT, M.DIV., SENIOR PASTOR

2004/2005 General Church Survey

Please answer the following questions.

1. What is your current age range?
A) 1-18
B) 19-29
C) 30-45
D) 46-56
E) 57-70
F) 71 or Higher

2. How did you come to be apart of the Jerusalem Baptist Church family?
A) Baptism
B) Letter form another church
C) Previous Christian Experience
D) Watchcare
E) Reinstatement of your membership from years ago.

3. How many church auxiliaries or ministries do you actively participate in?
A) One
B) Two
C) Three
D) Four
E) Five or more
F) None

4. List three (3) things that you value or like about your church home?
1._____
2._____
3._____

5. List three (3) things that you would change, modify, improve, or add to your church home?

1._____
2._____
3._____

APPENDIX H

HEALTH AWARENESS SERMON #1
"HE'S A KEEPER"

Sermon Series: "Health Awareness" Part I
"He's A Keeper"
I Thessalonians 5:23-24
Preached by: Pastor Michael Thomas Scott on Sun. March 5, 2006

My brothers and sisters, for the next few Sundays during the Lenten season, we will be observing a time of health awareness in the church. Now more than ever before, we are seeing a phenomenal rate of individuals that are "out-of-shape." Yes, "out-of-shape" physically, "out-of-shape" mentally, "out-of-shape" emotionally, and even "out-of shape spiritually! A well-noted Christian physician and author, Dr. Reginald Cherry, states that: "We as Americans spend more money on diet plans (Jenny Craig, Weight Watchers, Ultra Slim Fast), weight reduction programs, (Curves), pills, shots, and exercise equipment than the entire national budget of many countries. Isn't it ironic that with all of this money being spent, we as Americans in reality are still malnourished, overfed, obese, nutrient starved, sick and tired, tired and sick? Let me share with you, a week few weeks ago, I took a health survey, known as the "National Health Test", and I received the grade of "C" which is not that good because it means that I should be concerned about my health. I decided to bring the survey into the church and allow a few of our members to take it, only to discover, that I'm not the only one that needs to experience improvement in the area of health. I've learned that the majority of sick folk in this world are not in the hospitals, not in the nursing homes, not in convalescent centers. But there are more sick folk walking around here everyday and people don't even realize it. Some of these sick and out-of-shape people are right in your house, there at your place of employment, and God knows there even in the church. That was apart of the problem that the Apostle Paul was addressing in his letter/epistle to the church at Thessalonica.

This Thessalonian church had become somewhat "out-of-shape" because of the fact that they were so caught up in looking toward the future of the here and after, that they failed to be good stewards of everyday life in the here and now. They were so heavenly minded that they were doing themselves no earthly good. When Jesus said he was soon to return, they took him literally and they neglected the words of our Savior that states "He has come that we might have life and life more abundantly." My brothers and sisters, many of these church members had quit their jobs, because Jesus was coming back, packed their bags and stopped going to work, because Jesus was coming back, became freeloaders, because Jesus was coming back, neglected to handle their business, because Jesus was coming back, and sadly neglected to take care of their bodies, souls, and spirits because Jesus was coming back. Unfortunately, some of them forsook the faith, quit the church, became sexually promiscuous, engaged in disorderly conduct, became busybodies, and gossips, and the list goes on and on.

You know, good health is not just measured in blood pressure, sugar levels, and how much cholesterol you have. Good health is not just determined by the amount of push-ups, sit-ups, or jumping jacks that you can do. It doesn't really matter whether or not you run the 50-yard dash, 100-yard dash, or cross country. But are you in good shape with the Lord? Are you in good shape all the way around? Is your mind in good shape or do you say "sometimes I feel like a nut, and sometimes I don't?" Are your emotions in check or do you find yourself riding the roller coaster of life? Are you spiritually fit to fight the good fight of faith or do you feel like you've fallen and you can't get up? The question for most of us today, is not am I in good shape, because all of us can identify some area or areas in our lives that need to be shaped-up. But the question is how do I get in good shape all the way around? How can I be made whole? How can I get myself together?

Well, some folk will tell you, you need to lose some weight. Some folk will tell you, "you can start by eating the right foods." Some folk will tell you to get on the treadmill at the local (YMCA). Some folk will tell you to get some rest because "early to bed, early to rise, makes a man healthy, wealthy, and wise." Somebody might tell you eat your fruits and vegetables, "because an apple a day, keeps the doctor away." Some people will tell you to do this, that, and the other. But what does the text say? The Apostle Paul states in verse 23, "And the very God of peace sanctify you wholly..."

Understand, that we are unable to sanctify ourselves, only God can do that. We can't make ourselves whole, only God can do that. We should understand that the road to being kept, the road to health, the road to wellness and wholeness begins with God! And when we allow God to be first in all aspects of our lives, truly we can well-kept, truly we can be preserved, truly we can be what God desires us to be. If you give the Lord the opportunity to work in your life, scriptures declare that God will keep you.

Jude 1:24 states "Now unto Him that is able to keep you from falling and to present you faultless before the presence of his glory with exceeding joy..." God is able to keep you physically fit. The Message bible states that, "God is able to keep you on your feet!"

I'm looking at somebody that knows beyond a shadow of a doubt that God is able to keep you on your feet, because look at you right now! After all that you've been through....after all of your sickness and distress....heartaches and pains....sunshine and rain...after the dust has settled, you're still standing! God has kept you on your feet. Just when other thought that you would not make it, God kept you on your feet! Just when the enemy tried to rob you of your joy, your peace of mind, your praise, your testimony—God kept you on your feet! We serve a God that wants to be our keeper. God wants to keep you on your feet. God wants to keep you looking good and feeling good. Because when we look good and feel good, that makes God look good and feel good. God wants to keep you blessed. God will keep us on our feet.

Secondly, God wants to keep you mentally fit. The text indicates that we would be preserved blameless not only in body, but in the realm of the soul. The soul is the seat of the emotions, the mindset, the heart. The scriptures declare that "God will keep you in perfect peace whose mind is stayed in HIM! I don't know about you, but sometimes I need God to touch my mind, to keep me from going crazy. I need God to clothe me in my right mind! The seasoned saints had it right when they said, "I woke up this morning with my mind....stayed on Jesus, Halleliuah! God is a keeper of the mind. God is a keeper of the soul. God will keep you in perfect peace, if you let HIM!

Finally, God want to preserve your spirit. III John 1:2 states, "Beloved, I wish above all things that thou mayest proser and be in health, even as they soul prospers." We serve a God that wants us to healthy and whole all the way around, including our spiritual lives. God wants to keep us so that everything that we say and do will prosper. If we allow God to have His way in our lives and in our health, God will prosper us spiritually. He will bless us with every spiritual blessing in heavenly places in Christ Jesus! I don't know about you, but God is blessing me right now! He's keeping somebody right now! Somebody can testify that the reason why you are here this morning is because of the fact that God is keeping your spirit, God is blessing your spirit, God is encouraging your spirit to run on.

I am so glad that I serve a God that sent His son Jesus the Christ down through forty-two generations to save me, the heal me, to deliver me, and to make me whole again. I've tried Him and found out that He is a keeper! Have you tried Him for yourself? Do you know Him to be a keeper? It's not the Avon, Mary Kay, or Ebony Fashion Fair products keeping you---it's Jesus! It's not Hects, JCPenneys, or Peebles keeping you—it's Jesus. I've been in my prayer closet, had a little talk with Jesus! I've spent some time in the secret place of the Most High—it's Jesus! I've tried Him and found out, He's a keeper!

The hymnologist once wrote:
"Oh, to be kept by Jesus, Kept by the Power of God;
Kept from the world unspotted, treading where Jesus trod.
Oh, to be kept by Jesus, Lord at they feet I fall;
I would be nothing, nothing, nothing, Thou shalt be all in all!

Appendix I

Health Awareness Sermon #2
"Under New Management"

Sermon Series: "Health Awareness" Part II
"Under New Management"
I Corinthians 6:19-20
Preached by: Pastor Michael Thomas Scott on Sun. March 12, 2006

All throughout history, we have witnessed transition and transformation in politics, government, business, ministry, and particularly in corporate America. Many companies and corporations that were dying and suffering and on the verge of going down under had, enough sense to change administration. Something happened that should have caused a drastic turn-around for the better. About a year ago, my wife and I went to a certain restaurant chain in the Salisbury, Maryland area to get some pancakes. We were extremely dissatisfied with the service, the food, and atmosphere, and you name it…it was bad! To make a long story short, we decided that we would never ever go back to that restaurant again. I was talking to few other preachers in the neighborhood that had similar experiences with the same restaurant and they also stated, that they would not return. But one day, it just so happened that we had another taste or craving for pancakes and when we drove by this particular restaurant, there was a sign in front that said, "UNDER NEW MANAGEMENT." We decided to give it another try, and oh what a tremendous change for the better. I said all of that to say, that something ought to happen when leadership changes. Something ought to happen when the administration has shifted. Something ought to happen when under new management.

This principle of being under new management doesn't just apply to corporations, businesses, nations, and ministries, but this principle applies to people/individuals as well. As a matter of fact, the Apostle Paul pens this epistle, writes this letter, to the church at Corinth which was in similar situation. Paul is writing to this infantile church which he established some two or three years earlier. They were saved, but not yet fully delivered. They still had a some issues to work out in their lives. They were supposedly under new management, but some changes had not taken place. The Corinthian church was guilty of misrepresenting the Master, dishonoring the Divine, defrauding and defiling the Temple, and simply stated: they were giving the church a bad name! This was the church that had problems with sexual immorality, division, envy, strife, contention, and quarreling. This was the church were many were still sacrificing to idols and living foul lifestyles. Paul had to write to his church members to remind them that they were under new management.

Paul had to remind them and some of us to KNOW WHO WE ARE! The text states, "What! Know ye not that your body is the temple of the Holy Ghost?" Church we must understand, that when we give our lives over to the LORD JESUS, our bodies become "a living sacrifice." When we give ourselves to Christ, our bodies become temples of the Holy Ghost. Do you know who you are? You are a child of God. You are a King's kid. You are a "chosen generation, a royal priesthood, a holy nation." You are apart of the ekklessia—the generation that has been called out of darkness into the marvelous light! Do you know who you are? You are a representative of God here on the earth. You are an ambassador of God's kingdom. Do you know who you are? You are the temple of the Holy Ghost! Temple is defined as a sanctuary, holy place, a sacred place designated for the residence of a deity. Many people rise early on Sunday morning, eat their Sunday breakfast, put on the Sunday-go-to meeting clothes,

get in their Sunday morning automobile, put on the best "Sunday morning face," and state "I'm going to church." But when you know who you are, church takes on a deeper meaning. I'm no longer going to church, I am the church! When you know who you are, you realize and recognize that the church is in you! When you know who you are, you just can't live any kind of way. When you know who you are, you just can't eat how you want to eat. When you know that your body is the temple of God's Spirit, you can't put garbage into your system, because if you put garbage in, you'll get garbage out. When you know that your body is the temple of God's Spirit, you can't lay down with trash. If he or she won't put a ring on your finger, take them to the dump! God wants us to eat right, drink right, live right, and do right, because are bodies are His temples! Do you know who you are? You're walking around under new management. You've got Power in your body. You've got Authority in your body. You've got the Source of Life in your body. You've got the God of Abraham, Issac, Jacob…the God of Moses, Elisha, and David…the God of Peter, James, and John…in your body! Your song in the morning out to be:
"LORD, PREPARE ME TO BE A SANCTUARY, PURE AND HOLY, TRIED AND TRUE, AND WITH THANKSGIVING, I'LL BE A LIVING, SANCTUARY, LORD FOR YOU!"

The Apostle Paul reminds us that when you are under new management, you've got to KNOW WHOSE YOU ARE! The text states, "you are not your own; for you are bought with a price." The glorious good news of this text is that just when you where down so low, on your way to a devil's hell, there was a corporate take-over in heaven on your behalf. Just when your soul had gone into spiritual bankruptcy God sent his only begotten Son Jesus. You once were under the influence of the enemy. You once were a child of the devil, because we were all born and shapen in iniquity. But one day, God sent his Son, and the Son gave his life, paid the price in full on our behalf. You do know that the "wages of sin is death, but the gift of God is eternal life!" Do you know whose you are? You don't belong to the devil. You don't even belong to yourself. You belong to God. You've been bought with a price and now you're under new management. The adversary tried to use you up, to do his dirty work. The adversary tried to abuse your body with drugs and alcohol and you thought you were on top of the world until one day you woke up and the world was on top of you! The adversary had you thinking that sin was good for you. But now you realize that everything that may be good to you is not good for you! The good news is that now you are under new management.

Now that you're under new management, you're boss man has changed. Whose side are you leaning on, I'm leaning on the Lord's side. Now that you're under new management, your benefits have changed for the better: the Psalmist declares "Blessed be the Lord, who daily loadeth us with benefits, even the God of our salvation (Psalm 68:19)." "Bless the Lord, O my soul and forget not all his benefits: who forgives all thine iniquities, who heals all thy diseases, who redeems thy life from destruction; who crowns thee with lovingkindness and tender mercies; who satisfies thy mouth with good things, so that thy youth is renewed like the eagle's (Psalm 103: 1-5)."

Now that you're under new management, you're job description has changed. The text declares unto us what we are to do, "therefore GLORIFY God in your body, and in your spirit, which are the Lord's. Don't you know that I didn't come here this morning to look at my neighbor, I didn't come to study what you have on. But I came to glorify his name. Glorify, glorify, I come to magnify. I come to bless Him. I come to praise Him, because He's worthy. Isn't He worthy? He's good all the time! Every time I turn around, He keeps on blessing me! All I've got to do is glorify Him because I know He's alright!!! I'm under new management:

I've moved from my old house, I've moved from friends,
I've moved from my old way of life. Thank God I moved out, to a brand new life!
Can't you see that I'm a new man? Don't you know I've got a new name?
And one day, I'll live in a new land? Because I moved out to a brand new life!

Appendix J

Health Awareness Sermon #3
"Dealing With Depression"

Sermon Series: "Health Awareness" Part III
"Dealing With Depression"
Psalm 42:11

Preached by: Pastor Michael Thomas Scott on Sun. March 19, 2006

According to the National Institute of Mental Health, "depression strikes about 17 million adults in the United States of America each year—more than cancer, AIDS/HIV, or heart disease. Half of all Americans say they, or one of their family members, have suffered from depression." The Journal of the American Medical Association has stated "more suffering has resulted from depression than from any other single disease affection humankind." Depression can be mild or severe or somewhere in the middle. Depression can come in many forms or for many reasons. Depression could be linked to finances, employment, relationship, bereavement, grief, loss, or even birth. Have you ever been depressed about something and couldn't shake it off? Let's consider what our text says about depression this morning.

David, the great hero king of Israel and Judah, the Old Testament "prince of praise and worship"…David the "man after God's own heart", pens this didactic psalm while in a state of depression if you will. David pens this particular psalm what he was one the run. David pens this particular psalm at a time in his life where emptiness and darkness loomed all around him. His problems were piled a mile high. David had seemingly reached his own "personal ground zero." Have you ever been there church? You don't have to raise your hand. You don't have to say amen. Just blink your eyes. Sometimes our joy is depleted. Sometimes are hearts are heavy. Sometimes our soul is much discouraged. If we'll be honest with ourselves and honest with our God, all of us at one point in life have been in David's shoes. Can you remember feeling like your best days were actually behind you, even though folk were telling you that better days are ahead and the best is yet to come? Can you remember being in a room full of people, yet still feeling like you were alone, all by yourself, and discouraged? Have you ever had that emotional feeling that things would never improve in your life? Let me be the first to admit in this place, that I have been depressed before. Yes, the pastor of this great church. Depressed…with a robe! Depressed…with a collar! Depressed…with a bible in my hand! Yes, my brothers and sisters and you have been too. But the good news this morning is that you're not alone. As a matter of fact you're not the only one that have ever felt this way and you certainly won't be the last.

The prophet Elijiah was so depressed and downcast within his spirit that it was serious. After he had slain the prophets of Baal, that old wicked Queen Jezebel put a contract out on his life and she vowed that she would have him killed. Elijiah was being hunted down like an animal for doing the Lord's work. He was been sought after to be sifted out like wheat, for doing what was right in God's sight. The man of God found himself sitting underneath of a juniper tree and said "Lord, take my life."

Job, after Satan had afflicted him, caused him to lose his worldly possession. After Satan had stole from that which was dear to his heart. Job, my friends was so depressed that he cursed the very day that he was born.

Jeremiah, who wrote the book of Lamentation, was known to all as the "weeping prophet." He was so depressed that he said, I'm not going to tell it. I refuse to open my mouth. I'm not going to prophesy another word.

Paul, the Bible says had a thorn in his flesh, he asked the Lord to remove it three times to no avail.

Jesus, was depressed in the Garden of Gethsemane. The Bible declares that he was in agony and bitterness of soul. His spirit was so grieviously vexed that sweat as great drops of blood fell from his body onto the ground. Take courage today, you're not the first and certainly won't be the last. How do we deal with depression when it comes, because rest assured, it will eventually come your way? What did David do? How did David address this spiritual issues? David was cast down, disquieted, disturbed, but we see how he got over...

1. Keep Hope Alive. The Bible declares "hope thou in God". You know one thing that we should remember, is that there is always hope. No matter how dark and dismal the situation may seem to be. As long as there is breath in your body, there is always hope. Some of us need a little hope this morning, because hope in God is all that we have to keep us going. We've got to keep hope alive in our hearts. Keep hope alive in our minds. Keep hope alive in our souls. Keep hope alive that our blessing is right before us. Keep hope alive that our change is on the way. Keep hope alive that deliverance will come. To hope in God is to wait for something with confident and great expectation. Job said, "All the days of my appointed time, I'm going to wait for my change to come." Jeremiah, after going on strike , realized that there is something within, something on the inside, something going on

inside of me. It's just like fire, shut up in my bones! I just can't keep it to my self. Listen church, when the enemy of my life tries to depress my spirit, I have to keep hoping and trusting and believing that I've got the victory in the name of Jesus. When I begin to realize where all my help comes from I can muster up a praise to help me through my moment.

2. Have a Rehearsal. David said, "For I will yet praise Him. Hebrew translations of this verse seem to indicate that the psalmist was stating that I will praise Him over and over again till I get it in my spirit. I will praise Him over and over and over again until I remember. It's like having a rehearsal. You've got to go over it and over it again until you get down in your heart. So that when the enemy comes in. So that when troubles comes your way. So that when the depression is looming and darkness is glooming, you've got something in your heart. Remember the "joy of the Lord is your strength." This joy that we have, the world didn't give it and the world can't take it away. We've got to "rejoice in the Lord always, and again I say rejoice." Sometimes we throw words around in church so loosely, that oftentimes we miss the meaning of what we are saying. When the Bible says rejoice, "re" is the prefix and "joi" is the root word for joy. "RE" means to do something again as you did at first. So when the Bible tells us to rejoice, in essence, the Word is telling us that: whatever it took to get the joy…just do it again.

When you feel depressed in your spirit, just have a rehearsal. Praise God. Bless the Lord at all times, his praises shall continually be in my mouth! Just praise him in your own way! Just encourage yourself in the goodness of the Lord! What I like about this remedy, is that you can have a rehearsal anytime of the week, and hour of the day. You don't have to wait for choir practice. You don't have to wait for prayer service. You don't have to wait for Sunday morning. You can have a rehearsal in your car! You can have a rehearsal in the bathroom stall of your job. You can have a rehearsal in your kitchen. Just praise Him. Just bless Him. Just remember, reflect, recollect and rejoice in the fact that God has done great things. In everything give thanks for this is the will of God in Christ Jesus concerning you! It's not as bad as it seems. It could always be worse. Just thank God. Just praise God. Just bless His holy name. Because when praises go up…. the Blessor shows up! And when the blessor shows up…so

BIBLIOGRAPHY

Adams, Jay E. *Truth Applied*. Grand Rapids: Zondervan Publishing, 1990.

Anderson Bernhard W. *Understanding the Old Testament* 2nd edition. Englewood Cliffs, NJ: Prentice-Hall, 1966.

Arcury T.A., W.M. Gesier, and H.L. Cook. "Meaning in the Use of Unconventional Arthritis Therapies." *American Journal of Health Promotion* 14, no. 2 (February 1999): 78-85.

Ashing and K. Griva. "The recruitment of breast cancer survivors into cancer control studies; a focus on African-American women." *The Journal of the National Medical Association* (1999): 91,255-260.

Bailey, E.J. "Sociocultural factors and health-care seeking behaviors among Black Americans." *Journal of the National Medical Association* (1987): 79,389-392.

Blagrove, Sherine. "How Much Can the Safety Net Hold?" *Minority Health Today* (July 2000): 1.

Braaten, Carl E., ed. *Paul Tillich A History of Christian Thought: From Its Judaic and Hellenistic Origins to Existentialism*. New York: Simon and Schuster, 1968.

Briscoe V.J. and J.W. Pichert. "Promoting utilization of health care services through the African-American church." *The ABNF Journal* (1997): 7.

Brooks, Philip. *The Joy of Preaching*. Grand Rapids: Kregel Publications, 1989.

Brown, Raymond E. *An Introduction to the New Testament*. New York: Doubleday and Co. (1997).

Buttrick, David G. *Homiletic Moves and Structures*. Philadelphia: Fortress Press, (1987).

Campbel, Marci Kramish, et al. "Fruits and Vegetable Consumption and Prevention of Cancer: the Black Churches United for Better Health Project." *American Journal of Public Health* 89, no. 9 (1999): 1390-1396.

Cherry, Reginald Dr. *Healing Prayer: God's Divine Intervention in Medicine, Faith, and Prayer*. Nashville: Thomas Nelson Publishers, 1999.

Cheshire, Barbara W. *The Best Dissertation…A Finished Dissertation (Or Thesis)*. Portland, Oregon: National Book Company, 1993.

Claassens, L. Juliana M. *The God Who Provides: Biblical Images of Divine Nourishment*. Nashville: Abingdon Press, 2004.

Colbert, Don Dr. "Do you need Toxic Relief?" *Enjoying Everyday Life*, 2005, 22.

Coggins R.J. and J.L. Houlden, ed. *A Dictionary of Biblical Interpretation*. London: SCM Press, 1990.

Costen, Melva Wilson. *African American Christian Worship*. Nashville: Abingdon Press, 1993.

Covey, Stephen R. *The Seven Habits of Highly Effective People*. New York: Simon and Schuster, 1990.

Creswell, John W. *Research Design: Qualitative, Quantitative, and Mixed Methods Approaches* 2nd edition. Thousand Oaks: SAGE Publications, 2003.

Davis, C.M. and C.M. Curley. "Disparities of health in African-Americans." *Nursing Clinics of North America* (1999): 34,345-357.

Deffinbaugh, Bob. "Between a Rock and a Hard Place." [online]. Available from http://www.bible.org.

Drayton-Brooks, Shirlee. "Health promoting behaviors among African-American women with faith-based support." *The ABNF Journal* (September/October 2004).

Drayton-Hargrove, S. and J.H. Woods. "Ethical analysis of health care reform: Implications for diverse communities." *The ABNF Journal* (1995): 6, 99-103.

DuBois, W.E.B. *The Souls of Black Folk*. New York: Vintage Books, 1903.

Edge, Findley B. *The Doctrine of the Laity*. Nashville: Convention Press, 1985.

Epperly, Bruce G. and Lewis D. Solomon. *Walking in the Light: A Jewish-Christian Vision of Healing and Wholeness*. St. Louis: Chalice Press, 2004.

Erwin, D.O., T.S. Spatz, and R.C. Stotts, et al. "Increasing Mammography Practice among African-American Women." *Cancer Practice* 7, no. 2 (February 1999): 78-85.

Faull K., M. Hills, and G. Cochrane, et al. "Investigation of Health Perspectives of Those with Physical Disabilities: The Role of Spirituality as a Determinant of Health." *Disability Rehabilitation* 26, no. 3 (2004): 129-144.

Forbes, James. *The Holy Spirit and Preaching*. Nashville: Abingdon Press, 1989.

Gale, B.J. and J.R. Erickson. "How race affects health services use by older women." *Health Care for Women, International* (1997): 18, 221-232.

Gilbert, Rev. Richard B. ed. *Healthcare and Spirituality: Listening, Assessing, Caring.* Amityville, NY: Baywood Publishing Co., 2002.

Glanville C. and D. Porche. "Community level health promotion to improve the health status of African-Americans." *The Journal of Multicultural Nursing and Health* (1989): 4, 6-10.

Greenleaf, Robert K. *Servant Leadership.* New York: Paulist Press, 1997.

Greenwood, Davydd J. and Morten Levin. *An Introduction to Action Research: Social Research for Social Change.* Thousand Oaks: SAGE Publications, 1988.

Harris, James H. *Pastoral Theology: A Black Church Perspective.* Minneapolis: Fortress Press, 1991.

_____.*Preaching Liberation,* Minneapolis: Fortress Press, 1995.

_____. *The Word Made Plain: The Power and Promise of Preaching.* Minneapolis: Fortress Press, 2004.

Hartman, Louis F. and Alexander A. DiLella. *The Anchor Bible: The Book of Daniel* vol. 23. Garden City, NY: Doubleday and Co. Inc., 1978.

Haviland, William. *Cultural Anthropology.* Fort Worth: Harcourt Brace College Publishers, 1996.

Hodgson, Peter C. and Robert H. King. *Christian Theology: An Introduction to Its Traditions and Tasks.* Minneapolis: Fortress Press, 1994.

Horton-Brown, Hilary and Anjie Robsinson. "Healthy Habits are key to getting a hold on midterm stress." [Online]. Available from http://www.arbiteronline.com. November 2003.

Hover, Margot K. "Rural Clergy and Holistic Care." *Health Progress* (September/October 2005).

Jewell, John P. *Wired for Ministry: How the Internet, Visual Media, and Other New Technologies Can Serve Your Church.* Grand Rapids: Brazos Press, 2004.

Johnson-Cook, Susan. "'Breaking Traditions." *Gospel Today*, Volume 15 Issue 7, September/October 2004.

Jones, Miles J. *Preaching Papers: the Hampton and Virginia Union Lectures.* New York: Martin Luther King Fellows Press, 1995.

Jones, Tony. "Practical Theology," [online]. Available from http://www.theoblogy.blogspot.com.

Jung, Shannon. *Rural Ministry: The Shape of the Renewal to Come.* Nashville: Abingdon Press, 1998.

Kuntz, J. Kenneth. *The People of Ancient Israel: An Introduction to Old Testament Literature, History, and Thought.* New York: Harpers and Row Publishers, 1974.

Larimore, Walt. *Ten Essentials of Highly Healthy People.* Grand Rapids: Zondervan Press, 2003.

LaRue, Cleophus J. *The Heart of Black Preaching.* Louisville: Westminster John Knox Press, 2000.

Malkmus, George H. *Why Christians Get Sick.* Shippensburg, PA: Treasurer House, 1997.

Massey, James Earl. *The Responsible Pulpit.* Anderson, Indiana: Warner Press, 1974.

Maxwell, John C. *The 21 Indispensable Qualities of a Leader.* Nashville: Thomas Nelson Publishers, 1999.

Meier, August and Elliott Rudwick. *From Plantation to Ghetto* 3rd ed., New York: Hill and Wang, 1976.

Miller, Calvin. *Marketplace Preaching: How to Return the Sermon to Where it Belongs.* Grand Rapids, Baker Books, 1995.

Moyd, Olin P. *The Sacred Art.* Valley Forge: Judson Press, 1995.

Olitzky, Rabbi Kerry M. and Rabbi Daniel Judson. *The Rituals and Practices of Jewish Life: A Handbook for Personal Spiritual Renewal.* Woodstock, Vermont, Jewish Lights Publishing, 2002.

Olphen, Van, A. Schultz, B. Israel, L. Chatters, L. Klem, and D. Williams. "Religious involvement, social support and health among African-American women on the Eastside of Detroit." *Journal of General Internal Medicine* (2003): 18, 549-549-557.

Perry, John. *Unshakable Faith: Booker T. Washington & George Washington Carver.* Sisters, Oregon: Multnomah Publishers, 1999.

Perkins, John M. *Beyond Charity: The Call to Christian Community Development.* Grand Rapids: Baker Books, 1993.

_____. *Restoring At-Risk Communities: Doing It Together and Doing It Right.* Grand Rapids: Baker Books, 1995.

Phillips, J.B. *Letters to Young Churches: A translation of the New Testament Epistles.* New York: The MacMillan Co., 1961.

Pohly, Kenneth. *Transforming the Rough Places: The Ministry of Supervision.* Franklin, TN: Providence House Publishers, 2001.

Proctor, Samuel Dewitt. *The Substance of Things Hoped For: A Memoir of African-American Faith*. New York: G.P. Putnam's Sons, 1995.

Ramey, David A. *Empowering Leaders*. Kansas City: Sheed & Ward, 1991.

Rhein, Francis Bayard. *An Analytical Approach to the New Testament*. Woodbury, NY: Barron's Educational Services, Inc., 1996.

Roberts, Denton and Robert Hill. *Empowering Congregations: Successful Strategies for 21st Century Leadership*. Pasadena: Hope Publishing House, 2003.

Robinson, Haddon W. *Biblical Preaching: The Development and Delivery of Expository Messages*. Grand Rapids: Baker Books House, 1980.

Rubin, Jordan and David Remedios, M.D. *The Great Physician's Rx for Health and Wellness: Seven Keys to Unlock Your Health Potential*. Nashville: Thomas Nelson Publishers, 2005.

Schank M.J., D.Weiss, and R. Mathews. "Parish nursing: ministry of healing." *Geriatric Nursing* (1996): 17, 1-3.

Shawchuck, Norman and Roger Heuser. *Leading the Congregation: Caring for Yourself While Serving the People*. Nashville: Abingdon Press, 1993.

Stevenson, Dwight E. and Charles F. Diehl. *Reaching People from the Pulpit*. Grand Rapids: Baker Book House, 1958.

Stewart, Carlyle Fielding. *African American Church Growth: 12 Principles for Prophetic Ministry*. Nashville: Abingdon Press, 1994.

Stott, John R.W. *The Preachers' Portrait*. Grand Rapids: William B. Eerdmans Publishing Company, 1961.

Swears, Thomas. *Preaching to Head and Heart*. Nashville: Abingdon Press, 2000.

Taylor, Gardner C. *Chariots Aflame*. Nashville: Broadman Press, 1988.

Thomas, Frank A. *They Liked to Never Quit Praisin' God: The Role of Celebration in Preaching*. Cleveland: United Church Press, 1997.

Thomas, Terry Dr. *Becoming a Fruit-Bearing Disciple*. Raleigh, NC: Voice of Rehoboth Publishing, 2005.

Thompson, William D. *Preaching Biblically*. Nashville: Abingdon Press, 1981.

Turabian, Kate L. *A Manual for Writers of Term Papers, Theses, and Dissertations* 6th edition, Chicago: The University of Chicago Press, 1996.

U.S. Department of Health and Human Services. *Health Status of minorities and low income groups*. Washington D.C.: U.S. Government Printing Office, 1991.

_____. *Developing objectives for healthy people 2010*. Washington D.C.: U.S. Government Printing Office, 2002.

Unger, Merrill F. *The New Unger's Bible Dictionary*. Chicago: Moody Press, 1988.

Vine, W.E. *Vine's Complete Expository Dictionary of Old and New Testament Words*. Nashville: Thomas Nelson Publishers, 1985.

Vines, Jerry. *A Guide to Effective Sermon Delivery*. Chicago: Moody Press, 1986.

Visalli, Gayla ed. *After Jesus, The Triumph of Christianity.* Pleasantville, NY: Reader's Digest Association, Inc., 1992.

Walker, Wyatt T. *The Soul of Black Worship.* New York: Martin Luther King Fellows Press, 1984.

Wallis, Arthur. *God's Chosen Fast: A Spiritual and Practical Guide to Fasting.* Fort Washington, PA: Christian Literature Crusade, 1968.

Warren, Rick. *The Purpose Driven Life: What on Earth Am I Here For?* Grand Rapids: Zondervan Press, 2002.

Washington, Preston Robert. *God's Transforming Spirit: Black Church Renewal.* Valley Forge: Judson Press, 1988.

White, John. *Excellence in Leadership.* Downers Grove, Illinois: Inter-Varsity Press, 1986.